Our Nervous Friends

by Robert S. Carroll

A REMARK

Vividly as abstractions may be presented, they rarely succeed in revealing truths with the appealing intensity of living pictures. In Our Nervous Friends will be found portrayed, often with photographic clearness, a series of lives, with confidences protected, illustrating chapter for chapter the more vital principles of the author's The Mastery of Nervousness.

CHAPTER I

OUR FRIENDLY NERVES

"Hop up, Dick, love! See how glorious the sun is on the new snow. Now isn't that more beautiful than your dreams? And see the birdies! They can't find any breakfast. Let's hurry and have our morning wrestle and dress and give them some breakie before Anne calls."

The mother is Ethel Baxter Lord. She is thirty-eight, and Dick-boy is just five. The mother's face is striking, striking as an example of fine chiseling of features, each line standing for sensitiveness, and each change revealing refinement of thought. The eyes and hair are richly brown. Slender, graceful, perennially neat, she represents the mother beautiful, the wife inspiring, the friend beloved. Happily as we have seen her start a new day for Dick, did she always add some cheer, some fineness of touch, some joy of word, some stimulating helpfulness to every greeting, to every occasion.

The home was not pretentious. Thoroughly cozy, with many artistic touches within, it snuggled on the heights near Arlington, the close neighbor to many of the Nation's best memories, looking out on a noble sweep of the fine, old Potomac, with glimpses through the trees of the Nation's Capitol, glimpses revealing the best of its beauties. It was a home from which emanated an atmosphere of peace and repose which one seemed to feel even as one approached. It was a home pervaded with the breath of happiness, a home which none entered without benefit.

The husband, Martin Lord, was an expert chemist who had long been in the service of the Government. Capable, worthy, manly, he was blest in what he was, and in what he had. They had been married eight years, and the slipping away of the first child, Margaret, was the only sadness which had paused at their door. Mrs. Lord had been Ethel Baxter for thirty years. Her father was an intense, high-strung business man, an importer, who spent much time in Europe where he died of an American-contracted typhoid-fever, when Ethel was ten. Her mother was one of a large well-known Maryland family, fair, brown-eyed too, and frail; also, by all the rights of inheritance, training and development, sensitive and nervous. In her family the precedents of blue blood were religiously maintained with so much emphasis on the "blue" that no beginning was ever made in training her into a protective robustness. So, in spite of elaborate preparation and noted New York skill and the highest grade of conscientious nursing, she recovered poorly after Ethel's birth. Strength, even such as she formerly had, did not return. She didn't want to be an invalid. She was devoted to her husband and eager to companion and mother her child. The surgeons thought her recovery lay in their skill, and in ten years one operated twice, and two others operated once each, but for some reason the scalpel's edge did not reach the weakness. Then Mr. Baxter died, and all of her physical discomforts seemed intensified until, in desperation, the fifth operation was undertaken, which was long and severe, and from which she failed to react. So Ethel was an orphan at eleven, though not alone, for the good uncle, her mother's brother, took her to his home and never failed to respond to any impulse through which he felt he could fulfil the fatherhood and motherhood which he had assumed. Absolutely devoted, affectionate, emotional, he planned impulsively, he gave freely, but he knew not law nor order in his own high-keyed life; so neither law nor order entered into the training of his ward.

Ethel Baxter's childhood had been remarkably well influenced, considering the nervous intensity of both parents. For the mother's sake, their winters had been spent in Florida, their summers on Long Island. Her mother, in face of the fact that she rarely knew a day of physical comfort and for years had not felt the thrill of physical strength, most conscientiously gave time, thought and prayer to her child's rearing. Hours were devoted to daily lessons, and many habits of consideration and refinement, many ideals of beauty, many niceties of domestic duty and practically all her studies, were mother-taught. Ethel was active, physically restless, impulsive, cheerful, fairly intense in her eagerness for an expression of the thrilling activities within. She was truly a high-type product of generations of fine living, and her blue blood did show from the first in the rapid development of keenness of mind and acuteness of feeling. Typically of the nervous temperament, she early showed a superb capacity for complex adjustments. Yet, with one damaging, and later threatening idea, the mother infected the child's mind; the conception of invalidism entered into the constructive fabric of the child-thought all the more deeply, because there was little of offensively selfish invalidism ever displayed by the mother. But many of the concessions and considerations instinctively demanded by the nervous sufferer were for years matters-of-course in the Baxter home; and these demands, almost unconsciously made by the mother, could but modify much of the natural expression of her child's young years.

Another damaging attitude-reaction, intense in its expression, followed the unexpected death of Ethel's father. The mother, true to the ancient and honorable precedents of her family, went into a month of helplessness following the sad news. She could not attend the funeral, and for weeks the activities of the household were muffled by mourning; when she left her room, it was to wear the deepest crepe, while a half-inch of deadest black bordered the hundreds of responses which she personally sent to notes of condolence. She never spoke again of her husband without reference to her bereavement. Then, a year later, when the mother herself suddenly went, it seemed to devolve on the child to fulfil the mother's teachings. Her uncle's attitude, moreover, toward his sister's death was in many ways unhappy, for he did not repress expressions of bitterness toward the surgeons and condemned the fate which had so early robbed Ethel of both parents.

Thus, early and intensely, a morbid attitude toward death, a conviction that self-pity was reasonable, normal, wholesome, a belief that it was her duty to publicly display intensive evidences of her affliction, determined a lasting and potent influence in this girl's life which was to alloy her young womanhood-- disturbing factors, all, which before twelve caused much emotional disequilibrium. She now lived with her uncle in New York City and her summers were spent in Canada. The sense of fitness was so strong that during the next two vitally important, developing years she avoided any physical expression of her natural exuberance of spirits; and habits now formed which were, for years, to deny her any right use of her muscular self. She read much; she read well; she read intensely. She attended a private school and long before her time was an accredited young lady. Mentally, she matured very early, and with the exception of the damaging influences which have been mentioned, she represented a superior capacity for feeling and conceiving and accomplishing, even as she possessed an equally keen capacity for suffering.

She was most winsome at sixteen, a bit frail and fragile, often spoken of as a rare piece of Sevres, beloved with a tenderness which would have warped the disposition of one less unselfish; emotionally intense, brilliancy and vivacity periodically burst through the habit of her reserve. A perfect pupil, and in all fine things literary, keenly alive, she had written several short sketches which showed imaginative originality and a sympathetic sensitiveness, especially toward human suffering. And her uncle was sure that a greater than George Eliot had come. There was to be a year abroad, and as the doctor and her teacher in English agreed on Italy, there she went. At seventeen, during the year in Florence, the inevitable lover came. Family traditions, parents, her orphanage, the protective surroundings of her uncle's home, her instincts--all had kept her apart. Her knowledge of young lovers was but literary, and this particular young lover presented a side which soon laid deep hold on her confidence. They studied Italian together. He was musical, she was poetic, and he gracefully fitted her sonnets to melodies. Finally, it seemed that the great Song of Life had brought them together to complete one of its harmonies. Her confidence grew to love, the love which seemed to stand to her for life. Then the awful suddenness, which had in the past marked her sorrows, burst in again. In one heart-breaking, repelling half-hour his other self was revealed, and a damaged love was left to minister to wretchedness. Here was a hurt denied even the expression of mourning stationery or black apparel--a hurt which must be hidden and ever crowded back into the bursting within. Immediate catastrophe would probably have followed had not, first, the fine pride of her fine self, then the demands of her art for expression, stepped in to save. She would write. She now knew human nature. She had tasted bitterness; and with renewed seriousness she became a severely hard- working student. But the wealth of her joy-life slipped away; the morbid made itself apparent in every chapter she wrote, while intensity became more and more the key-note of thought and effort.

Back at her uncle's home, the uncle who was now even more convinced that Ethel had never outlived the shock of the loss of her parents, she found that honest study and devotion to her self-imposed tasks, and a life of much physical comfort and rarely artistic surroundings, were all failing to make living worth while. In fact, things were getting into a tangle. She was becoming noticeably restless. Repose was so lost that it was only with increasing effort that she could avoid attracting the attention of those near. Even in church it would seem that some demon of unrest would never be appeased and only could be satisfied by constant changing of position. Thoughts of father and mother, and the affair in Florence, intensified this spirit of unrest, and few conscious minutes passed that unseen stray locks were not being replaced. It seemed to be a relief to take off and put on, time and again, the ring which had been her mother's. Even her feet seemed to rebel at the confinement of shoes, and she became obsessed with the impulse to remove them, even in the theater or at the concert. A sighing habit developed. It had been growing for years into an air- hunger, and finally all physical, and much of mental, effort developed a sense of suffocation which demanded short periods of absolute rest. Associations were then formed between certain foods and disturbing digestive sensations. Tea alone seemed to help, and she became dependent upon increasingly numerous cups of this beverage. Knowing her history as we do, we can easily see how she had become abnormally acute in her responses to the discomforts which are always associated with painful emotions, and that emotional distress was interpreted, or misinterpreted, as physical disorder. Each year she became more truly a sensitive-plant, suffering and keenly alive to every discomfort, more and more easily fatigued by the conflicts between emotions, which craved expression, and the will, which demanded repression.

Since the days in Florence there had been a growing antagonism to men, certainly to all who indicated any suitor-like attitude. In her heart she was forsworn. She had loved deeply once. Her idealism said it could never come again. But her antagonism, and her idealism, and her strength of will all failed to satisfy an inarticulate something which locked her in her room for hours of repressed, unexplained sobbing. Her writing became exhausting. Talks before her literary class were a nightmare of anticipation--for through all, there had never been any weakening of the beauty and intensity of her unselfish desire to give to the world her best. The dear old uncle watched her with growing apprehension. He persuaded her to seek health. It was first a water- cure; then a minor, but ineffective operation; then much scientific massage; and finally a rest-cure, and at the end no relief that lasted, but a recurrence of symptoms which, to the uncle, spoke ominously of a threatened mental balance. What truly was wrong? Do we not see that this woman's nerves were crying out for help; that, as her wisest friends, they were appealing for right ways of living; that they were pleading for development of the body that had been only half-trained; that they were beseeching a replacing of morbidness of feeling by those lost joyous happiness-days? Were they not fairly cursing the wrong which had robbed her of the hope and rights of her womanhood?

A new life came when she was twenty-eight, with the saving helper who heard the cry of the suffering nerves, and interpreted their message. She had told him all. His wise kindness made it easy to tell all. He showed her the wrong invalidism thoughts, the unhappy, depressing, devitalizing attitude toward death. He revealed truths unthought by her of manhood and womanhood. He pointed out the poisonous trail of her enmity, and she put it from her. He inspired her to make friends with her nerves, who were so devotedly striving to save her. Simple, definite counsel he gave, for her body's sake. Her physical development could never be what early constructive care would have made it, but from out of her frailty grew, in less than a year of active building-training, a reserve of strength unknown for generations in the women of her line. Wholesome advice made her see the undermining influence of her morbid, mental habits, and resolutely she displaced them with the productive kind that builds character. Finally, new wisdom and a truly womanly conception of her duty and privilege replaced her antagonism to men, as understanding had obliterated enmity. It would seem as though Providence had been only waiting these changes, for they had hardly become certainties in her life when the real lover came--a man in every way worthy her fineness of instinct; one who could understand her literary ambitions and even helpfully criticize her work; one who brought wholesome habits of life and thought, and who could return cheer for cheer, and whose love responded in kind to that which now so wonderfully welled up within her.

Her new adjustments were to be deeply tried and their solidity and worthiness tested to their center. Little Margaret came to make their rare home perfect, and like a choice flower, she thrived in the glow of its sunshine. At eighteen months, she was an ideal of babyhood. Then the infection from an unknown source, the treacherous scarlatina, the days of fierce, losing conflict, and sudden Death again smote Ethel Lord. But she now knew and understood. There was deep sadness of loss; there was greater joy in having had. There was an emptiness where the little life had called forth loving attention; there was a fulness of perfect mother-love which could never be taken. There were no funeral days, no mourning black, no gruesome burial. There were flowers, more tender love, and a beautified sorrow. Death was never again to stand to Ethel Lord as irreparable loss, for a great faith had made such loss impossible.

And such is the life of this woman, filled with the spirit of beauty of soul--a woman who thrills husband and son with the uplift of her unremitting joy in living, who inspires uncle and friends as one who has mastered the art of a happy life, who holds the devotion of neighbors and servants through her unselfish radiation of cheer. Ethel Lord has learned truly the infinitely rich possibilities of our nerves when we make them our friends.

CHAPTER II

THE NEUROTIC

For four heart-breaking years, the strife of a nation at war with itself had spread desolation and sorrow broadcast. The fighting ceased in April. One mid-June day following, the town folk and those from countrysides far and near met on the ample grounds of a bride-to-be. Had it not been for the sprinkling of blue uniforms, no thought of war could have seemed possible that fair day. The bride's home had been a-bustle with weeks of preparation for this hour, and nature was rejoicing and the heavens smiling upon the occasion. Sam Clayton, the bridegroom, was certainly a "lucky dog." A quiet, unobtrusive son of a neighboring farmer, he and Elizabeth had been school-children together. Probably the war had lessened her opportunity for choice but the night before he left for the front, they were engaged--and her family was the best and wealthiest of the county. "Lucky dog" and "war romance," the men said. Nevertheless, six weeks ago he had returned with his chevrons well-earned, and fifty years of square living later proved his unquestioned worth. Elizabeth at twenty, on her bridal day, was slender, lithe, fair-skinned; of Scotch-Irish descent, her gray eyes bespoke her efficiency--to-day, they spoke her pride, though neither to-day nor in years to come were they often softened by love. But it was a great wedding, and the eating and dancing and merry- making continued late into the night with ample hospitality through the morrow for the many who had come far. "Perfectly suited," the women said of the young couple.

Sam Clayton had nothing which could be discounted at the bank, but the bride was given fifty fertile acres, and they both had industry and thrift, ambition and pluck. The fifty acres blossomed--Sam was a good farmer, but he proved himself a better trader, and before many years was running a small store in town. They soon added other fifty acres-- one-hundred-and-fifty in fifteen years, and out of debt--then a partner with money, and a thriving business. At forty-five it was: Mr. Samuel Clayton, President of the Farmers' and Merchants' Bank, rated at $150,000. Mrs. Clayton's ability had early been manifest. Before her marriage she had taken prizes at the County Fair in crocheting and plum-jell. In after years no one pretended to compete with her annual exhibit of canned fruits, and the coveted prize to the County's best butter-maker was awarded her many successive autumns.

Our real interest in the Claytons must begin twenty-five years after the happy wedding. Their town, the county seat, had pushed its limits to the skirts of the broad Clayton acres; theirs was now the leading family in that section. Mr. Clayton, quiet, active, practical, was capable of adjusting himself without disturbance to whatever conditions he met. Three children had been born during the early years--a girl and two younger boys. The daughter was of the father's type--reserved, studious and truly worthy, for during the years that were to come, with the man she loved waiting, she remained at home a pillar of strength to which her mother clung. She turned from wifehood in response to the selfish needs of this mother. She and the older brother finished classical courses in the near-by "University," for their mother, particularly, believed in education. The brother and sister had much in common, were indeed much alike; he, however, soon married and moved into the new West and deservingly prospered. Fred, the youngest, was different. During his second summer he was very ill with cholera infantum-- the days came and went--doctors came and went-- and the wonder was how life clung to the emaciated form. The mother's love flamed forth with intensity and the nights without sleep multiplied until she, too, looked wan and ill. She did not know how to pray. Her parents had been Universalists-- she termed herself a Moralist; for her, heaven held no God that can hear, no Great Heart that cares, no Understanding that notes a mother's agony. The doctors offered no hope. The child was starving; no food nor medicine had agreed, and the end was near. A neighboring grandmother told how her child had been sick the same way, and how she had given him baked sweet potato which was the first thing he had digested for days. As fate would have it, it was even so with Fred, and he recovered leaving his mother devoid of faith in any one calling himself doctor, and fanatically devoted to the child she had so nearly lost. From that sickness she hovered over him, protecting him from the training she gave her other children--the kind she herself had received. His wish became her law; he was humored into weakness. He never became robust physically, and early showed defects quite unknown in either branch of the family. He failed in college, for which failure his mother found adequate excuse. He entered the bank, but within a few months his peculations would have been discovered had he not confessed to his mother, who made the discrepancy good from her private funds. During the next few years she found it necessary on repeated occasions to draw cheeks on her personal account to save him from trouble--but never a word of censure for him, always excuses. He was drinking, those days, and gambling. In the near-by state capitol the cards went his way one night. Hilarious with success and drink, he started for his room. There was a mix-up with his companions. He was left in the snow, unconscious--his winnings gone. The wealth of his father and the devotion of his mother could not save him, and he went with pneumonia a few days later. It was said that this caused her breakdown--let us see.

As a girl, Elizabeth had lived in a home of plenty, in a home of local aristocracy. She was perfectly trained in all household activities and, for that period, had an excellent education, having spent one year in a far-away "Female Seminary." Her mind was good, her pride in appearance almost excessive. She said she "loved Sam Clayton," and probably did, though with none of the devotion she gave her son, nor with sufficient trust to share her patrimony which amounted to a small fortune with him when it came. In fact, she ran her own business, nor relied upon the safety of the "Farmers' and Merchants' Bank" in making her deposits. She was a housewife of repute, devoted to every detail of housewifery and economics. There was always plenty to eat and of the best; perfect order and cleanliness of the immaculate type were her pride. Excellent advice she frequently gave her husband about finances and management, but otherwise she added no interest to his life, and there was peace between husband and wife--because Sam was a peaceable man. As a mother, she taught the two older children domestic usefulness, with every care; they were always clad in good, clean clothes, clad better than the neighbors' children, and education was made to take first rank in their minds. Her sense of duty to them was strong; she frequently said: "I live and save and slave for my children." Fred, as we have seen, was her weakness. For him she broke every rule and law of her life.

At forty-five she was thin, her face already deeply seamed with worry lines, a veritable slave to her home, but an autocrat to servants, agents and merchants. They said her will was strong; at least, excepting Fred, she had never been known to give in to any one. We have not spoken of Mary. Poor woman! She, too, was a slave--she was the hired girl. Meek almost to automatism, a machine which never varied from one year's end to another, faithful as the proverbial dog, she noiselessly slipped through her unceasing round of duties for twenty-three years--then catastrophe. "That fool hired man has hoodwinked Mary." No wedding gift, no note of well-wishing, but a rabid bundling out of her effects. Howbeit, Central Ohio could not produce another Mary, and from then on a new interest was added to the Claytons' table-talk as one servant followed another into the Mother's bad graces. She was already worn to a feather-edge before Mary's ingratitude. But the shock of Fred's death completed the demoralization of wrongly lived years. For weeks she railed at a society which did not protect its citizens, at a church which failed to make men good, while she now recognized a God against whom she could express resentment.

This woman endowed with an excellent physical and mental organization had allowed her ability and capacity to become perverted. Orderliness, at first a well planned daily routine, gradually degenerated into an obsession for cleanliness. Each piece of furniture went through its weekly polishing, rugs were swept and dusted, sponged and sunned--even Mary could not do the table-linen to her taste--and Tuesday afternoon through the years went to immaculate ironing. The obsession for cleanliness bred a fear of uncleanliness, and for years each dish was examined by reflected light, to be condemned by one least streak. The milk and butter especially must receive care equaled only by surgical asepsis. Then there were the doors. The front door was for company, and then only for the elect--and Fred; the side door was for the family, and woe to the neighbor's child or the green delivery boy who tracked mud through this portal. No amount of foot-wiping could render the hired man fit for the kitchen steps after milking time--he used a step-ladder to bring up the milk to the back porch. Such intensity of attention to detail could not long fail to make this degenerating neurotic take note of her own body, which gradually became more and more sensitive, till she was fairly distraught between her fear of draughts and her mania for ventilation. It was windows up and windows down, opening the dampers and closing the dampers, something for her shoulders and more fresh air. Church, lecture-halls and theaters gradually became impossible. Finally she was practically a prisoner in the semiobscurity of her home--a prisoner to bodily sensation. Then came the autos to curse. The Clayton home was within a hundred yards of the county road, and when the wind was from the west really visible dust from passing motors presumed to invade the sanctity of parlor and spare rooms, and with kindling resentment windows were closed and windows were opened, rooms were dusted and redusted until she hated the sound of an auto-horn, until the smell of burning gasoline caused her nausea--but each year the autos multiplied.

At last the family realized that her loss of control was becoming serious, that she was really a sufferer; but her antagonism to physicians was deep-set, so the osteopath was called. Had he been given a fair chance, he might have helped, but her obsessions were such that she resented the touch of his manipulations, fearing that some unknown infection might exude from his palms to her undoing. Reason finally became helpless in the grip of her phobias. Her stomach lining was "destroyed," and into this "raw stomach" only the rarest of foods and those of her own preparation could be taken. She had fainted at Fred's funeral, and repeatedly became dazed, practically unconscious, at the mention of his name. Self-interests had held her attention from girlhood to her wreckage, and from this grew self- study, which later degenerated into self-pity. Her converse was of food and feelings and self. She bored all she met, for self alone was expressed in actions and words.

Father and daughter finally, under the pretext of a trip for her health, placed her in a Southern sanitarium. Much was done here for her, in the face of her protest. Illustrative of the unreasoning intensity with which fear had laid hold upon her was her mortal dread of grape-seeds. As she was again being taught to eat rationally, grapes were ordered for her morning meal. The nurse noticed that with painful care she separated each seed from the pulp, and explained to her the value of grape-seeds in her case. She wisely did not argue with the nurse, but two mornings later she was discovered ejecting and secreting the seeds. The physician then kindly and earnestly appealed for her intelligent cooperation. She thereupon admitted that many years ago a neighbor's boy had died of appendicitis, which the doctor said was caused by a grape-seed. The fallacy of these early-day opinions was shown her. Then was illustrated the weakness of her faith and the strength of her fear. She produced a draft for one thousand dollars, which she said she always carried for unforeseen emergencies, and offered it to the doctor to use for charity or as he wished, if he would change the order about the grapes. Suffice it to say she learned to eat Concords, Catawbas, Tokays and Malagas. She returned home better, but was never wholesomely well, and to-day dreads the death for which her family wait with unconscious patience.

What is the secret of this miserable old woman's failure to adjust herself to the richness which life offered her? A selfish self peers out from every act. Even her generosity to Fred was the pleasing of self. Given all that she had, what could she not have been! Physically, with the advantages of plenty and her country life and the promise of her fair girlhood, what attraction could not have been hers had kindness and generosity softened her eyes, tinted her cheeks, and love-wrinkles come instead of worry-wrinkles.

Her mind was naturally an unusual one. She lived within driving distance of one of Ohio's largest colleges--only an hour by train to the state capital. Fortune had truly smiled and selected her for happiness, but from the first it was self or her family and no further thought or plan or consideration.

Elizabeth Clayton was given a nervous system of superb quality, which used for the good of those she touched would have hallowed her life; misused, she drifts into unlovable old age, a selfish neurotic. She could have been a leader in her community, a blessing in her generation, a builder of faiths which do not die, but she failed to choose the good part which neither loss of servant, death of child nor advancing age can take away.

CHAPTER III

THE PRICE OF NERVOUSNESS

The price we pay for defective nerves is one of mankind's big burdens. Humanity reaches its vaunted supremacy, it realizes the heights of manhood and womanhood through its power to meet what the day brings, to collect the best therefrom and to fit itself profitably to use that best for the good of its kind. And these possibilities are all dependent on the superb, complicated nervous system. The miracles of right and wise living are rooted deep in the nerve-centers. Man's nervous system is his adjusting mechanism--his indicator revealing the proper methods of reaction. Nothing man will ever make can rival its sensitiveness and capacity. But when it is out of order, trouble is certain. Excessive, imperfect, inadequate reactions will occur and disintegrating forms of response to ourselves and our surroundings will certainly become habitual, unless wise and resolute readjustments are made. The common failure of the many to find the best, even the good in life, is apparent to all--so common indeed, that the search for the perfectly adjusted man, physically, mentally, morally adjusted, is about as fruitful as Diogenes' daylight excursions with his lantern. The physical, mental and moral are intricately related even as the primary colors in the rainbow. Our nerves enter intimately into every feeling, thought, act of life, into every function of our bodies, into every aspiration of our souls. They determine our digestion and our destinies; they may even influence the destinies of others. Let us turn a few pages of a life and see the cost of defective nervous-living.

The Pullman was crowded; every berth had been sold; the train was loaded with holiday travelers, and the ever interesting bridal couple had the drawing-room. The aisle was cluttered with valises and suitcases; the porter was feverishly making down a berth; while bolstered on a pile of pillows, surrounded by a number of anxious faces, lay the sick woman, the source of the commotion and the anxiety. Sobs followed groans, and exclamations followed sobs-- apparently only an intense effort of self-control kept her from screaming. She held her head. Periodically, it seemed to relieve her to tear at her hair. She held her breath, she clutched her throat, she covered her eyes as though she would shut out every glimpse of life. She convulsively pressed her heart to keep it from bursting through; she clasped and wrung her hands, and now and then would crowd her forearm between her teeth to shut in her pent-up anguish. She would have thrown herself from the seat but for the unobtrusive little man who knelt in front to keep her from falling, and gently held her on as she spasmodically writhed. His plain, unromantic face showed deep anxiety, not unmixed with fear. He was eagerly assisted by the dear old lady who sat in front. Hers was mother-heart clear through; her satchel had been disturbed to the depths in her search for remedies long faithful in alleviating ministration; her camphor bottle lay on the floor, impulsively struck from her kind hand by the convulsed woman. The sweet-faced college girl who sat opposite had just finished a year in physiology and this was her first opportunity to use her new knowledge. "Loosen her collar and lower her head and let her have more air," she advised. "Yes," said the little man, "I'm her husband you see, and am a doctor. I've seen her this way before and those things don't help."

The drummer, who had the upper berth, had retreated at the first sign of trouble to the safety of the smoking-room, and was apparently trying more completely to hide himself in clouds of obscuring cigar smoke. The passengers were all cowed into attentive quietude; the sympathetic had offered their help, while the others found satisfaction for their aloofness in agreement with the sophisticated porter, who, after he had assisted in safely depositing the writhing woman behind the green curtains and had been rather roughly treated by her protesting heels, shrewdly opined to the smoking-room refugees that "That woman sho has one case o' high-strikes." The berth, however, proved no panacea--she was "suffocating," she must get out of the smoke and dust, she must get away from "those people" or she would stifle, and to the other symptoms were added paroxysms of coughing and gasping which sent shivers through the whole car of her sympathizers. Her husband explained that she was just out of a hospital, which they had left unexpectedly for home, that she never could sleep in a berth, and if they could only get the drawing-room so he could be alone with her he thought he could get her to sleep, but he did not know what the consequences would be if she did not get quiet. The Pullman conductor was strong for quiet, and he and the sweet-faced college girl and the dear old lady formed a committee who waited on the young bride and groom. It was hard, mighty hard, even in the bliss of their happiness, to give up the drawing-room for a lower. Had not that drawing-room stood out as one of their precious dreams during the last year, as, step by step, they had planned in anticipation of that short bridal week! But the sacrifice was made, the transfers effected, and out of the quiet which followed, emerged order and the cheer normal to holiday travelers. A number were gratified by the sense of their well- doing, they had gone their limit to help; others were equally comfortable in their satisfied sense of shrewdness, they agreed with the porter--they had sized her up and not been "taken in."

Mrs. Platt had been Lena Dalton. She was born in Galveston forty-five years before. Her father was a cattle-buyer, rough, dissipated, always indulgent to himself and, when mellow with drink, lavishly indulgent to the family. He never crossed Lena; even when sober and irritable to the rest, she had her way with him. The high point in his moral life was reached when she was seven. For three weeks she was desperately ill. A noted revivalist was filling a large tent twice a day; the father attended. He promised himself to join the church if Lena did not die--she got well, so there was no need. She remained his favorite. "Drunk man's luck" forgot him several years later when his pony fell and rolled on him, breaking more ribs than could be mended. He left some insurance, two daughters, and a very efficient widow. Mrs. Dalton had held her own with her husband, even when he was at his worst. She was strong of body and mind, practical, probably somewhat hard, certainly with no sympathy for folderols. Her common-school education, in the country, had not opened many vistas in theories and ideals, but she lived her narrow life well, doing as she would be done by--which was not asking much, nor giving much--caring for herself without fear or favor till she died, as she wished, at night alone, when she was eighty. She possessed qualities which with the help of a normal husband would have been a wholesome heritage to the children; but it was a home of double standards, certainly so in the training of Lena, who had never failed, when her father was home, to get the things her mother had denied her in his absence. She was thirteen when he died; at fifteen then followed her two most normal years. The accident occurred which, was to prove fateful for her life, and through hers, for others.

Lena was a good roller-skater, but was upset one night, at the rink, by an awkward novice and fell sharply on the back of her head. She was taken home unconscious and was afterward delirious, not being herself until noon the next day, when she found beside her an anxious mother who for several days continued ministering to her daughter's every wish. Three months later she set her heart on a certain dress in a near-by shop window; her mother said it was too old for her, and cost too much. Day after day passed and the dress remained there, more to be desired each time she saw it. The Sunday-school picnic was only a week off. She made another appeal at the supper table; her sister unwisely interjected a sympathetic "too bad." The emphasis of the mother's "No" sounded like a "settler," but just then things went dark for Lena. She grasped her head and apparently was about to fall--her face twitched and her body jerked convulsively. The mother lost her nerve, and feeling that her harshness had brought back the "brain symptoms" which followed the skating accident, spent the night in ministrations--and hanging at the foot of Lena's bed, when she was herself next morning, was the coveted dress. To those who know, the mental processes were simple; strong desire, an implacable mother, save when touched by maternal fear, the association in the girl's mind of a relationship between her accident and her mother's compliance, a remoter association of her illness at seven with her father's years of free giving. What was to restrain her jerkings and twitchings and meanings? Many of these reactions were taking place in the semi-mysterious laboratory of her subconscious self; but it was the beginning of a life of periodic outbreaks through which she had practically never failed to secure what she desired. To the end of her good mother's life, Lena remained the only one who could change her "no" to "yes."

The elder sister was a more normal girl. She studied stenography and soon married a promising young man. They had two children. He made a trip down the coast and died of yellow fever. The wife was much depressed and spent a bad year and most of the insurance money, getting adjusted. Then the Galveston storm with its harvest of death and miraculous escapes--the mother was taken, the two children left. Meanwhile Lena had finished high school, had taken a year in the Normal and secured a community school to teach, near Houston. She was now eighteen, her face was interesting, some of the features were fine. Her bluish-gray eyes could be particularly appealing;

there was much mobility of expression; a wealth of slightly curling, light-chestnut hair was always stylishly arranged; in fact, her whole make- up caused the young fellows to speak of her as the "cityfied school- marm." Then came the merchant's son and all was going well, so well that they both pledged their love and plighted their troth. The temporary distraction of her lover's attention, deflected by the visiting brunette in silks, an inadvertently broken appointment (the train was late and he could not help it), and the first attack of the "jerks" among strangers is recorded. They hastily summoned old Jake Platt's son, just fresh from medical college, who, helpless with this suffering bit of femininity, supplied in attention and practical nursing what he lacked in medical discernment and skill, to the end that one engagement was broken and another formed in a fortnight. Old Jake had some money; the young doctor was starting in well, and needed a wife; she was still jealous, and young Dr. Platt got a wife, who molded his future as the modeler does his clay.

Within the first month the bride had another attack. They had planned a trip to Houston to do some shopping and to attend the theater. The doctor-husband was delayed on a case and found his young bride in the throes of another nervous storm when he reached home, nor did the symptoms entirely abate until he had promised her that he would always come at once, no matter what other duties he might have, when she needed him. By this promise he handicapped his future success as a physician and did all that devoted ignorance could do to make certain a periodic repetition of the convulsive seizures. This was but the first of a series of concessions which involved his professional, social and financial future, which her "infirmity" exacted of him as the years passed. Later old Jake died and the doctor's share of his big farms was an opportune help. But Mrs. Platt had a certain far-reaching ambition; therefore, they soon moved to Houston. He would have done well where he started; his education, his medical equipment, his personality were certain to limit his progress in a city. The doctor's wife was superficially bright, capable of adapting herself with distinct charm to those she admired. She formed intense likes and dislikes--while often impulsively kind-hearted, she could cling to vindictive abuse for months. Here was a woman who proved very useful on church committees, in societies, in Sunday-school, who worked effectively in the Civic Club. She sang fairly well naturally, of course "adored music" and was an efficient enthusiastic worker when interested. But Lena Platt was never able to work when not interested.

Periodically her "fearful nervous spells" would interfere with all duties. The doctor was absolutely subsidized. Had any other attractions appealed to him, his wife's early evidences of implacable jealousy would have proven a sure antidote. He was an unconscious slave. Her nervousness expressed itself toward him in other terms than convulsively. She had a tongue which from time to time blistered the poor man. He would never talk back, fearful as he ever was of bringing on one of those storms which, in his inadequate medical knowledge, were as mysterious and ominous as epileptic attacks.

For years the absence of children in the home was a sorrow from which much affecting sentimentality evolved, being as well the pathetic cause for days of sickness, when outside interests were less attractive to this artful sufferer than the attentions elicited by her illness. Then out of the great gulf surged the heroic Galveston tragedy, and the two orphan children came to fill the idealized want. At first they received an abundance of impulsive loving, but unhappily one day, a few months after they came, the foster-mother overheard the elder girl make an unfavorable comparison between her and the real mother; and for years distinctions were made--the younger being always favored, the unfortunate, older child living half-terrorized, never knowing when angry, unfair words would assail her.

Lena Platt had confided to several of her bosom friends the tragedy of her unequal marriage and that she knew she would yet find a "soul mate." There was a Choral Society in Houston one winter, and following a few gratuitous compliments from the dapper young director, she decided she had found it. He left in the spring and this dream faded. A few months later the new minister's incautious exaggeration that "he didn't know how he could run the church without her" came near resulting in trouble, for some of the good sisters unkindly questioned the quality of her sudden excessive devotion and religious zeal. Mrs. Platt was not vicious, but she craved excitement; hers was a life of constantly forming new plans. Attention from any source was sweet and from those of prominence it was nectar. Things were pretty bad in the doctor's home after the preacher episode, and she was finally persuaded to let her husband call in another physician. He was very nice to her, and while he never pretended to understand her case, his medicine and advice benefited her tremendously and she went nearly a year without a bad attack. Her visits to his office and her conscienceless use of his time were finally brought to a sudden close when one day he deliberately called other patients in, leaving her unnoticed in the waiting-room. Bad times again, then other new doctors, other periods of immunity from attacks, with exaggerated devotion to each new helper until she had made the rounds of the desirable, professional talent of Houston.

Meanwhile, impulsive extravagance had sadly reduced the Platt inheritance, so when an acquaintance returned from St. Louis nervously recreated by a specialist there, the poor doctor had to borrow on his insurance to make it possible for her to have the benefit of this noted physician's skill. The trip North meant sacrifice for the entire family. Apparently she wished to be cured, and the treatment began most auspiciously. After careful, expert investigation, assurance had been given that if she would do her part, she could be made well in six months. Her husband told the physician that he hoped he would "look in on her often, for she will do anything on earth for one she likes." The treatment was thorough-going; it began at the beginning, and during the early weeks she was enthusiastically satisfied with the skill of her treatment and the care of her special nurse, in whom she found another "bosom friend," to whom she confided all. Her devotion for the new doctor grew by leaps. Mistaking his kindness and thinking perchance she might extract more beneficent sympathy by physical methods, she impulsively threw herself into where-his-arms-would-have- been had he not side-stepped. Her position physically and sentimentally was awkward; the doctor called the nurse and left her. Later he returned and did his best to appeal to her womanhood; he analyzed her illness and showed her some of the damage it had wrought both in her character and to others. He showed her the demoralization which had grown out of her wretched surrender to impulsive desire. He revealed to her the necessity for the effacement of much of her false self and the true spiritualizing of her mind as the only road to wholesome living. That same day Dr. Platt received a telegram peremptorily demanding that he come for her. Upon his arrival he had a short talk with the specialist who succinctly told him the problem as he saw it. For a few minutes, and for a few minutes only, was his faith in the helpless reality of his wife's sickness shaken; but faith and pity and indignation were united as she told of her mistreatment and how she had been outraged and her whole character questioned by that "brutal doctor," who talked to her as no one had ever dared before. She was going home on the first train and going home we found her, having another attack in the Pullman. A collapse, her husband told himself, from over-exertion and the result of her wounded womanhood. "A plain case o' high-strikes" was the porter's diagnosis; a sickness sufficiently adequate to have the sweet incense of much public attention poured upon her wounded spirit--and to secure the coveted drawing-room!

On her way home! She had spurned her one chance to be scientifically taught the woefully needed lessons of right living-on her way to the home which had become more and more chaotic with the passing of the years and the dwindling of their means.

Who can count the price this woman has paid for her nervousness? At fifty, with a scrawny, under-nourished body, the wrinkled remnants of beauty, she suffers actual weakness and distress. Quick prostration follows all effort, excepting when she is fired by excitement. All ability to reason in the face of desire is gone; she is dominated by emotions which become each year more unattractive; even the air- castles are tumbled into ruins. Her husband is a slave--used as a convenience. Her waning best is for those who attract her, her growing worst for those who offend. One child's life is maimed by indulgence, the other's by injustice. She has reached that moral depravity which fails to recognize and accept any truth which is opposed to her wishes. As she looks back over the vista of years, filled with many activities, no monument of wholesome constructiveness remains; she has blighted what she touched. Lena Platt, a wilful, spoiled, selfish hysteric!

CHAPTER IV

WRECKING A GENERATION

The afternoon's heat was intense; it was reflecting in shimmering waves from everything motionless, this breathless September day in Donaldsville, Texas. Main Street is a half-mile long, unpainted "box- houses" fringe either end and cluster unkemptly to the west, forming the "city's" thickly populated "darky town." Near the station stands the new three-story brick hotel, the pride of the metropolis. Not even the Court House at the county seat is as imposing. Main Street is flanked by parallel rows of one and two story, brick store-buildings, from the fronts of which, and covering the wide, board-sidewalks, extend permanent, wooden awnings; these are bordered by long racks used for the ponies and mules of the Saturday crowds of "bottom niggers" and "post oak farmers." The higher ground east of Main Street is preempted by the comfortable residences of Donaldsville proper and culminates in Quality Hill, where the two bankers and a select group of wealthy bottom-planters lived in aristocratic supremacy. On this particular afternoon, the town's only business street was about deserted. On its shady side were hitched a few Texas ponies whose drooping heads and wilted ears bespoke the heat--so hot it was that the flies, even, did not molest them. Scattered groups of lounging, idle men indicated the enervating influence of the sizzling 108 degrees in the shade.

But Donaldsville was not dead--perspiring certainly, but still possessing one lively evidence of animation. From time to time peals of boisterous laughter, boisterous but refreshing as the breath of a breeze, a congenial, almost contagious laughter would roll up and down Main Street even to its box-house fringes. Each peal would call forth from some dusky denizen of the suburbs the proud recognition: "Dar's Doctor Jim laughin' some mo'." Doctor Jim's laughter was one of Donaldsville's attractive features. His friends living a mile away claimed they often heard it--and everybody was Doctor Jim's friend. No more genial, generous gentleman of the early post-bellum Texas South could be found. His was an unfathomed well of good nature, good humor and good stories. He knew all comers whether he had met them before or not. For him, it was never "Stranger," it was always "Friend."

Let us take his proffered hand and feel the heartiness of its greeting, feel its friendly shake, even to our shoe-soles. His good humor beams from his deep-blue eyes; his shock of gray hair, which knows no comb but his fingers, is pushed back from a brow which might have been a scholar's, were it not so florid. A soft, white linen shirt rolls deeply open, exposing a grizzled expanse of powerful chest. Roomy, baggy, spotless, linen trousers do homage to the heat, as does his broad, palm-fiber hat, used chiefly as a fan. Doctor Jim McDonald, six feet in his socks, weighing 180 pounds, erect and manly in bearing in spite of his negligee, is a remarkable specimen of physical manhood at sixty-five. Even with the Saturday afternoon crowds of the cotton-picking season, Main Street seems deserted if his resounding laughter is not heard; but it takes something as serious as a funeral to keep him away from his accustomed bench in front of Doctor Will's drug-store, centrally located on the shady side of the street. Doctor Will is Doctor Jim's brother, and is, according to the negroes, a "sho-nuff" doctor.

Doctor Jim's life is comfortably monotonous. He had put up the first windmill in the region roundabout and his was the first real bath-tub in the county, and long before Donaldsville thought of water-works, Doctor Jim's windmill was keeping the big cistern on stilts filled from his deep artesian well. He started each day with a stimulating plunge in his big tub, and never tired proclaiming that with this and enough good whiskey he would live to be a hundred--and then Main Street would stop and listen to the generous reverberations of his deep-chested laugh. Three good meals, the best old Aunt Sue could cook and Aunt Sue came from Mississippi with them after the war--were eaten with an unflagging relish by this man whose digestion had never discovered itself. Two mornings a week Doctor Jim drove leisurely out to his big Trinity River plantation, a two-thousand-acre plantation, where he was the beloved overlord of sixty negro families. This rich, river-bottom farm, when cotton was at a good price, brought in so much that Doctor Jim, with another of his big laughs, would say he was "mighty lucky in having those rascally twins to throw some of it away." One night a week he could always be found at the Lodge, and once a day he covered each way the half-mile separating his generous, rambling home on Quality Hill and Doctor Will's office. His only real recreation was funerals. He would desert his shady seat and drive miles to help lay away friend or foe--if foes he had. On such occasions only, would he pass the threshold of a church. He contributed generously to each of the town's five denominations and showed considerable restraint in the presence of the cloth in his choice of reminiscences, but it was always the occasion of a good- natured uproar for him to proclaim, "The Missus has enough religion for us both." Still the silence of his charity could have said truly that his donation had constructed one-fifth of each church-building in the town; in fact, it was his pride to double the Biblical one-tenth in his giving.

Of his open-heartedness Doctor Jim rarely spoke but another pride was his, to which he allowed no day to pass without some hilariously expressed reference. He was proud of his whiskey-drinking. One quart of Kentucky's best Bourbon from sun to sun, decade after decade! "I have drunk enough whiskey to float a ship--and some ship too. Look at me! Where will you find a healthier man at sixty-five? I haven't known a sick minute since the war. If you drink whiskey right, with plenty of water and plenty of eatin', it won't hurt anybody." This was the law and the gospel to Doctor Jim; he never failed to proclaim it to pale-faced youths or ailing mankind; and the Book of

Judgment, alone, will reveal the harvest of destruction which Time reaped through Doctor Jim's influence in L---County. Yet, oddly, it was Doctor Jim's principle and practice never to treat. He claimed he had never offered a living soul a social drink.

"Drink whiskey right and it won't hurt anybody!" Did it hurt?

Doctor Jim and his two brothers spent their early life on a plantation in Mississippi. The father wanted the boys to be educated. Two of them took medical courses in New Orleans. Doctor Jim wished to see more of the world, and literally did see much of it on a two-year cruise around the Horn to the East Indies and China. He was thirty-five years old in '60 when he married. Then he served as surgeon--"mighty poor surgeon" he used to say, for a Mississippi regiment throughout the four years of the Civil War. He and his two brothers passed through this conflict and returned home to find their father dead, the negroes scattered and the old plantation devastated. The three with their families journeyed to Texas--the then Land of Promise! At twenty-five cents an acre they bought river-bottom lands which are to-day priceless, and the losses of the past were soon forgotten in the rapid prosperity of the following years.

Mrs. McDonald represented all that high type of character which the dark years of the war brought out in so many instances of Southern womanhood. Patient, hopeful, uncomplaining she lived through the four years of war-time separation, left her own people and journeyed to the Southwest to begin life anew. She was particularly robust of physique, domestic in a high sense, gentle and deeply kind. She passed through hardship, privation and prosperity practically not knowing sickness. Her children could not have had better mother-stock, and the scant days were in the past, so they never knew the lack of plenty. There were eight, from Edith, born in 1870, to Frank, in 1885, including the twins.

Did whiskey-drinking hurt?

Edith grew into a slender, retiring girl, her paleness accentuated by her black hair. She was quiet, read much, and took little interest in out-of-door activities, entering into the play-life of the other children but rarely. Her father insisted, later, on her riding, and she became a fair horsewoman. She was refined in all her relations. Edith went to New Orleans at seventeen. The spring after, she developed a hacking cough and had one or two slight hemorrhages, but at twenty was better and married an excellent young merchant. The child was born when she was twenty-two; three weeks later the mother died, leaving a pitiable, scrofulous baby, which medical and nursing skill kept lingering eighteen months.

The first boy was named James, Jr., as we should expect, and, as we should not expect, was never called "Jim." But James was not right. He developed slowly, did not walk till over three, was talking poorly at five; he was subject to convulsions and destructive outbreaks; he was uncertain and clumsy in his movements, so provision was made that he might always have some one with him. But even in the face of this care, he stumbled and fell into the laundry-pot with its boiling family-wash, was badly scalded and seriously blinded. James mercifully died two years later in one of his convulsions.

Mabel was the flower of the family. Through her girlhood she was lovable in every way, and beloved. She was blond like her father, though not as robust as either father or mother, and in ideals and character was truly the latter's daughter. She finished in a finishing school, had musical ability and charm, and soon married and made a happy home--an unusual home, until the birth of the first child. Since then it has been a fight for health, with the pall of her family's history smothering each rekindling hope. Operations and sanatoria, health-resorts and specialists have not restored, and she lives, a neurasthenic mother of two neurotic children. Happiness has long fled the home where it so loved to bide those early days, before the strain and stress of maternity had drained the mother's poor reserve of vitality.

The history of Will and John, named for the two uncles, would prove racy reading through many chapters. "The Twins" were the father's text for spicy stories galore many years before their death. From the first, they were "two young sinners." They both had active minds-- overactive in devising deviltry. Mischievous as little fellows, never punished, practically never corrected by their father, humored by sisters, house-servants, and the plantation-hands, feared and admired by other boys, they seemed proof against any helpful influence from the earnest, pained, prayerful mother. As boys of ten, they had become "town talk" and were held responsible for all pranks and practical jokes perpetrated in Donaldsville or thereabout, unless other guilty ones were captured red-handed. Multiply your conception of a "bad boy" by two and you will have Will at twelve; repeat the process and you will have John. They possessed one quality--dare we call it virtue?-- which kept them dear to Doctor Jim's heart through their very worst. They never lied to him, no matter what their misdeeds. They could lie as veritable troopers, but from him the truth in its rankest boldness was never withheld. As the years passed, they made many and deep excursions into the old doctor's pocket. But he paid the bills cheerfully and sent his reverberating laugh chasing the speedy dollars, as soon as he got with some of his Main Street cronies. The boys planned and worked together, protecting each other most cleverly. Still they were expelled from every school they attended after they were thirteen. A military academy noted for its ability to handle hard cases found them quite too mature in their wild ways, and sent them home. They may, for reasons best known to themselves, have been "square with the old man," but they were a pair of thoroughgoing toughs by twenty, not only fast but cruel, even brutal, in their evil- doing.

Will was the first to show the strain of the pace. When twenty-two, the warning cough sobered him a bit, and in John's faithful and congenial company, he went first to Denver, then to New Mexico. Doctors' orders were irksome, whiskey and cards the only available recreation for the boys, and so they tried to follow their father's example in developing a powerful physique on Kentucky Bourbon ("best"). John suddenly quit drinking. "Acute nephritis" was on the shipping paster. Delirium tremens was the truth. Will was too frail to accompany his brother's remains home. He was pretty lonely and anxious, and miserable without John, but for several weeks behaved quite to the doctor's satisfaction. It didn't last long, and within the year tuberculosis and Bourbon laid him beside his brother.

May was a promising girl, "almost a hoiden," the neighbors said. She rode the ponies bareback; she played boys' games, and at twelve looked as though the problem of health could never complicate her glad, young life. But cough and hemorrhage, twin specters, stalked in at sixteen and the poor child fairly melted away and was gone in a year.

Annabel, the youngest girl, was a quiet child and thoughtful. Some called her dull, but rather, it seems, she early sensed her fate. When but a child she was sent to "San Antone" and operated on by a throat specialist. After May's death she went to the mountains each summer and spent two winters in South Texas. But she grew more and more thin, and in the end it was tuberculosis.

Frank, the last child, was different from all the others. He seemed bright of mind and active of body. He attended school as had none of the other boys; he even went to Sunday-school. Physically and mentally, he gave promise of prolonging the family line--but he proved his father's only admitted regret. He lied and he stole. The money which his father would have given him freely he preferred to get by cunning. Doctor Jim could not tolerate what he called dishonesty, and from time to time they would have words and Frank would be gone for months. His cleverness made him a fairly successful gambler; that he played the game "crooked" is probably evidenced by his being shot in a gambling-joint before he was thirty.

We have thus scanned the-wreckage of a generation bred in alcohol. Children they were of unusual physical and mental parentage, parents who never knowingly offended their consciences, children reared in most healthful surroundings with every comfort and opportunity for normal development. Four of them showed their physical inferiority through the early infection and unusually poor resistance to tuberculosis; one was born an imbecile; one died directly from the effects of drink; the only girl who survived early maturity, the best of them all, spent twenty years a nervous sufferer, mothering two nervously defective children; the physically best was the morally worst and died a criminal.

Doctor Jim lived on with his habits unchanged, his laugh, only, losing something in volume and more in infectiousness. Still proud of his health he preached the gospel of good whiskey well drunk, never sensing his part in the tragedy of his own fireside. He was nearly eighty when the stroke came which bereft him of any possibility of understanding, or of knowing remorse. He had laid his wife away some years previously and for months he lingered on paralyzed, demented, in the big, empty house, cared for by an old negro couple, hardly recognizing Mabel when she came twice a year, but never forgetting that, "Whiskey won't hurt anybody."

CHAPTER V

THE NERVOUSLY DAMAGED MOTHER

His name is not Lawrence Adams Abbott. The surname really is that of one of America's first families. He, himself, is among the few living of a third generation of large wealth.

It was an early-summer afternoon and Dr. Abbott--for he was a graduate of Cornell Medical--was standing at one of the train gates of the Grand Central Station in New York. As he waits apart from the small crowd assembled to welcome, he attracts observing attention. His face appears thirty; he is thirty-six. The features are finely cut, the chin is especially good. The eyes are blue-gray, and a slight pallor probably adds to his apparent distinction. His attitude is languid, the handling of his cane gracefully indolent, the almost habitual twisting of his chestnut-brown mustache attractively self-satisfied. His clothing is handsome, of distinctive materials, and tailored to the day. So much for an observing estimate. The critical observer would note more. He would detect a sluggishness in the responses of the pupils, as the eyes listlessly travel from face to face, producing an effect of haunting dulness. Mumbling movements of the lips, a slightly incoordinate swaying of the body, might speak for short periods of more than absent-mindedness.

But the gates open and after the eager, intense meetings, and the more matter-of-fact assumption of babies and bundles, the red-capped porters, with their lucky burdens of fashionable traveling-cases, pilot or follow the sirs and mesdames of fortune. Among these is one whose handsome face is mellowed by softening, early-gray hair, and whose perfect attire and tenderness in greeting our doctor at once associate mother and son. She has just come down the Hudson on one of the few seriously difficult errands of her fifty-six years.

Two weeks have passed. The room is stark bare, save for two mattresses, a heap of disheveled bed clothes, and two men. The hours are small and the dim, guarded light, intended to soften, probably intensifies the weirdness of the picture. The suspiciously plain woodwork is enameled in a dull monochrome. The windows are guarded with protecting screens. One man, an attendant, lies orderly on his pallet; the other, a slender figure in pajamas, crouches in a corner. His hair is bestraggled; his face is livid; his pupils, widely dilated; his dry lips part now and then as he mutters and mumbles inarticulately or chuckles inanely. Now starting, again abstracted, he is capable of responding for a moment only, as the attendant offers him his nourishment. A few seconds later he is groaning and twisting, obviously in pain, pain which is forgotten as quickly, as he reaches here and there for imaginary, flying, floating things. Real sleep has not closed his eyes for now nearly three nights. He is delirious in an artificial, merciful semi-stupor, which is saving him the untold sufferings of morphine denial. Before this unhappy Dr. Abbott stretch long, wearisome weeks of readjustment, weeks of physical pain and mental discomfort, weeks, let us hope, of soul-prodding remorse. His only chance for a future worth spending lies in months of physical reeducation, of teaching his femininely soft body the hardness which stands for manliness; for him must be multiplied days of mental reorganization to change the will of a weakling into saving masterfulness; nor will these suffice unless, in the white heat of a moral revelation, the false tinsel woven into the fabric of his character be consumed. For months he must deny himself the luxuries, even many of the comforts, his mother's wealth is eager to give. Yet these weeks and months of development may never be, for in a short time he will again be legally accountable, and probably will resent and refuse constructive discipline, and return to a satin-upholstered life--his cigarettes, his wine-dinners, his liquors, and his "rotten feeling" mornings after--then to his morphin and to his certain degradation. And why should this be? Time must turn back the hands on her dial thirty-three years that we may know.

The fine Abbott home was surrounded by a small suburban estate near Philadelphia, a generation ago; we have met the then young mistress of the mansion, at the Grand Central Station. It was a home of richness, a home of discriminating wealth, a home of artistic beauty; it was a home of nervous tension. This neurotic intensity was not of the cheap helter-skelter, melodramatic sort; there was a splendid veneer of control. But all the mother's plans and activities depended on the moods, whims and impulses of little Lawrence, the only child, then glorying in the hey-day of his three-year-old babyhood. It was a household kept in dignified turmoil by this child of wealth, who needed a poor boy's chance to be a lovable, hearty, normal chap. It was overattention to his health, with its hundreds of impending possibilities; to his food, with the unsolvable perplexity of what the doctor advised and of what the young sire wanted. More of satisfaction, perhaps, was found in clothing the youth, as he cared less about these details; still, an unending variety of weights and materials was provided that all hygienic and social requirements might be adequately met. Anxious thought was daily spent that his play and playmates might be equally pleasing and free from danger. Almost prayerful investigation was made of the servants who ministered, and tense, sleepless hours were spent by this nervous mother striving to wisely decide between the dangers to her child of travel and those other dangers of heated summers and bleak winters at home. Frequent trips into the city and frequent visitations from the city were made, that expert advice be obtained. Consultations were followed by counter consultations and conferences which but added the mocking counsel of indecision. And the marble of her beauty began to show faint marrings chiseled by tension and anxiety--for was not Lawrence her only son!

It was a home of double standards. The father was a wholesome, serious-minded, essentially reasonable, Cornell man. His ideas were manly and from time to time he laid down certain principles, and when at home, with apparently little effort, exacted and secured a ready and certainly not unhappy, obedience from his son. But business interests and responsibilities were large and the bracing tonic of his association with the boy was all too passing to put much blood- richness into the pallor of the child's developing character. Moreover, this intermittent helpfulness was more than counteracted by the mother's disloyal, though unconscious dishonesty. Hers was an open, if need be a furtive, overattention and overstimulation, an inveterate surrender to the sweet tyranny of her son's childish whims. There was probably nothing malicious in her many little plans which kept the father out of the nursery and ignorant of much of their boy's tutelage. The mother was only repeating fully in principle, and largely in detail, her own rearing; and had she not "turned out to be one of the favored few?"

The suburban special went into a crash, and all that a fine father might have done through future years to neutralize the unwholesome training of a nervous mother was lost. In fact, her power for harm was now multiplied. The large properties and business were hers through life, and with husband gone, and so tragically, there was increased opportunity, and unquestionably more reason, for the intensification of her motherly care. So the fate of a fine man's son is left in the hands of a servile mother.

It now became a home of restrained extravagance. The table was fairly smothered with rare and rich foods. Fine wines and imported liquors entered into sauces and seasonings. The boy's playroom was a veritable toy-shop, with its hundreds of useless and unused playthings. Long before any capacity for understanding enjoyment had come, this unfortunate child had lost all love for the simple. With Mrs. Abbott, it was always "the best that money can buy"--unwittingly, the worst for her child's character. It was a home of formal morality. Sunday morning services were religiously attended; charities of free giving, the giving which did not cost personal effort, were never failing. It was a home of selfish unselfishness. All weaknesses in the son throughout the passing years were winked at. Never from his mother did Lawrence know that sympathy, sometimes hard, often abrupt, never pampering, which breeds self-help.

Lawrence went to the most painstakingly selected, private preparatory-schools, and later, as good Abbotts had done for generations, entered Cornell. He had no taste for business. For years he had been associated with gifted and agreeable doctors; he liked the dignity of the title; so, after two years of academic work, he entered the medical department and graduated with his class. These were good years. His was not a nature of active evil. Many of his impulses were quite wholesome, and college fraternity camaraderie brought out much that was worthy. In the face of maternal anxiety and protest, he went out for track, made good, stuck to his training and in his senior year represented the scarlet and white, getting a second in the intercollegiate low hurdles. Another trolley crash now, and he might have been saved!

All through his college days a morbid fear had shortened his mother's sleep hours with its wretchedness. Her boy was everything that would attract attractive women. Away from her influence he might marry beneath him, so all the refinements of intrigue and diplomacy were utilized that a certain daughter of blood and wealth might become her daughter-in-law. The two women were clever, and woe it was that his commencement-day was soon followed by his wedding-day. No more sumptuous wedding-trip could have been arranged-to California, to the Islands of the Pacific, to India, to Egypt, then a comfortable meandering through Europe. A year of joy-living they planned that they might learn to know each other, with all the ministers of happiness in attendance. But the disagreements of two petted children made murky many a day of their prolonged festal journey, and beclouded for them both many days of the elaborate home-making after the home-coming. And the murkiness and cloudiness were not dissipated when parenthood was theirs. Neither had learned the first page in Life's text-book of happiness, and as both, could not have their way at the same time, rifts grew into chasms which widened and deepened. Then the wife sought attentions she did not get at home in social circles and the husband sought comforts his wife and his home did not give, in drink and fast living, later with cocain and morphin. The ugliness of it all could not be lessened by the divorce, which became inevitable. By mutual agreement, the rearing of the child was intrusted to the father's mother, who to-day shapes its destiny with the same unwholesome solicitude which denied to her own son the heritage of wholesome living.

We met father and grandmother as she arrived in New York to arrange for the treatment, which even his beclouded brain recognized as urgent; and we leave him with a darkening future, unless Fate snatches away a great family's millions, or works the miracle of self- revelation, or the greater miracle of late-life reformation in the son of this nervously damaged mother.

CHAPTER VI

THE MESS OF POTTAGE

"I know Clara puts too much butter in her fudge. It always gives me a splitting headache, but gee, isn't it good! I couldn't help eating it if I knew it was going to kill me the next day." The Pale Girl looks the truth of her exclamations, as she strolls down the campus-walk arm-in-arm with the Brown Girl, between lectures the morning after.

Clara Denny had given the "Solemn Circle" another of her swell fudge- feasts in her room the night before, and, as usual, had wrecked sleep, breakfast, and morning recitations for the elect half-dozen, with the very richness of her hand-brewed lusciousness. They called Clara the Buxom Lass, and they called her well. She was, physically, a mature young woman at sixteen, healthy, vigorous, rose-cheeked, plump, and not uncomely, frolicsome and care-free, with ten dollars a week, "just for fun." She was a worthy leader of the Solemn Circle of sophomores which she had organized, each member of which was sacredly sworn to meet every Friday night for one superb hour of savory sumptuousness-- in the vernacular, "swell feeds."

Clara was a Floridian. Her father had shrewdly monopolized the transfer business in the state's metropolis, and from an humble one- horse start now operated two-score moving-vans and motor-trucks, and added substantially, each year, to his real-estate holdings. Mr. Denny let fall an Irish syllable from time to time, regularly took his little "nip o' spirits," and ate proverbially long and often. Year after year passed, with the hardy man a literal cheer-leader in the Denny household, till his gradually hardening arteries began to leak. Then came the change which brought Clara home from college--home, first to companion, then to nurse, and finally through ugly years, to slave for this disintegrating remnant of humanity. Slowly, reluctantly, this genial, old soul descended the scale of human life. He was dear and pathetic in the early, unaccustomed awkwardness of his painless weakness. "Only a few days, darlin', and we'll have a spin in the car and your father'll show thim upstarts how to rustle up the business." The rustling days did not come, but short periods of irritability did. He wanted his "Clara-girl" near and became impatient in her absence. He objected to her mother's nursing, and later became suspicious that she was conspiring to keep Clara from him, and often greeted both mother and daughter with unreasonable words. His interests narrowed pitiably, until they did not extend beyond the range of his senses, and the senses themselves dulled, even as did his feelings of fineness. He grew careless in his habits, and required increasing attention to his beard and clothing. Coarseness first peeped in, then became a permanent guest--a coarseness which the wife's presence seemed to inflame, and which could be stilled finally only by the actual caress of his daughter's lips. And with the slow melting of brain-tissue went every vestige of decency; vile thoughts which had never crossed the threshold of John Denny's normal mind seemed bred without restraint in the caldron of his diseased brain. His was a vital sturdiness which, for ten years, refused death, but during the last of these he was physically and morally repellent. Sentiment, that too-often fear of unkind gossip, or ignorant falsifying of consequences, stood between this family and the proper institutional and professional care, which could have given him more than any family's love, and protected those who had their lives to live from memories which are mercilessly cruel.

Clara's older brother had much of his father's good cheer and less of his father's good sense. He, too, had money to use "just for fun," and Jacksonville was very wide open. So, after his father's misfortune had eliminated paternal restraint, the boy's "nips o' spirits" multiplied into full half-pints. For twelve years he drank badly, was cursed by his father, prayed for by his mother, and wept over by Clara. The wonderful power of a Christian revival saved him. He "got religion" and got it right, and lives a sane, sober life.

The older sister had married while Clara was at school, and lived with her little family in Charleston. Her "duty" was in her home, but this duty became strikingly emphasized when things "went wrong" in Jacksonville, and she frankly admitted that she was entirely "too nervous to be of any use around sickness"; nor did she ever come to help, even when Clara's cup of trouble seemed running over. And this cup was filled with bitterness when, suddenly, the mother had a "stroke," and the care of two invalids and the presence of her periodically drunk brother made ruthless demands on her twenty years. The mother had been a sensible woman, for her advantages, and most efficient, and under her teaching Clara had become exceptionally capable. The two invalids now lay in adjoining rooms. "Either one may go at any time," the doctor said, and when alone in the house with them the daughter was haunted with a morbid dread which frequently caused her to hesitate before opening the door, with the fear that she might find a parent gone. As it happened, she was away, taking treatment, unable to return home, when grippe and pneumonia took the mother, and the candle of the father's life finally flickered out.

Clara had handled the home situation with intermittent efficiency. When she entered her father's sick-room, called suddenly from the thoughtless hilarities of the Solemn Circle and fudge-feasts, and saw him so altered, and, for him, so dangerously frail, in his invalid chair, something went wrong with her breathing; the air could not get into her lungs; there was a smothering in her throat and she toppled over on the bed. It seemed to take smelling-salts and brandy to bring her back. She said afterwards that she was not unconscious, that she knew all that was happening, but felt a stifling sense of suffocation. Later after one of her father's first unnatural outbreaks, she suffered a series of chills and her mother thought, of course, it was malaria; but many big doses of quinin did not break it up, and no matter when the doctor came, his little thermometer revealed no fever. She spent three months at Old Point Comfort and the chills were never so bad again. Other distressing internal symptoms appeared closely following the shock of her mother's sudden paralysis. An operation and a month in a northern hospital were followed by comparative relief. But her nervous symptoms finally became acute and she was spending the spring and early summer on rest-cure in a sanitarium when her parents died. The Jacksonville home was then closed.

Soon after, Clara was profoundly impressed at the same revival in which her brother was converted. While she could not leave her church to join this less formal denomination, she entered into Home Missionary activities with much zest. At this time a friendship was formed with a woman-physician who, as months of association passed, attained a reasonably clear insight into her life and encouraged her to enter a well-equipped, church training-school for deaconesses. The spell of the religious influences of the past year's revival was still strong; this, and the stimulation of new resolves, carried her along well for six months. In her studies and practical work she showed ability, efficiency and flashes of common sense. Then she became enamored of a younger woman, a class-mate--her heart was empty and hungry for the love which means so much to woman's life. Unhappily, she overheard her unfaithful loved one comment to a confidante: "It makes me sick to be kissed by Clara Denny." Another damaging shock, followed by another series of bad attacks--the old spells, chills and internal revolutions had returned. She rapidly became useless and a burden. The school-doctor sent her a thousand miles to another specialist.

We first met Clara Denny effervescent, winning, almost charming--a sixteen-year-old minx. Let us scrutinize her at thirty-six. What a deformation! She weighs one hundred and seventy-three--she is only five-feet-four; her face is heavy, soggy, vapid; her eyes, abnormally small; her complexion is sallow, almost muddy; her chin, trembling and double; strongly penciled, black eye-brows are the only remnant apparent of the "Buxom Lass" of twenty years ago. Her hands are pudgy; her figure soft, mushy, sloppy; her presence is unwholesome. The specialist found her internally as she appeared externally. While not organically diseased, the vital organs were functionally inert. Every physical and chemical evidence pointed to the accumulation in a naturally robust body of the twin toxins--food poison and under oxidation. She was haunted by a fear of paralysis. She confused feelings with ideas and was certain her mind was going. The spells which had first started beside her invalid father were now of daily occurrence. She, nor any one else knew when she would topple over. She found another reason for her belief that her brain was affected in her increasingly frequent headaches. For years she had been unable to read or study without her glasses, because of the pain at the base of her brain. When these wonderful glasses were tested, they were found to represent one of the mildest corrections made by opticians; in fact, her eyes were above the average. Her precious glasses were practically window-glass.

Much of each day had been spent in bed, and hot coffee and hot-water bottles were required to keep off the nerve-racking chills which otherwise followed each fainting spell. Her appetite never flagged. She had been a heavy meat eater from childhood. There never was a Denny meal without at least two kinds of meat, and one cup of coffee always, more frequently two-- no namby-pamby Postum effects, but the genuine "black-drip." In the face of much dental work, her sweet tooth had never been filled. She loved food, and her appetite demanded quantity as well as quality. Of peculiar significance was the fact that throughout the years she had never had a spell when physically and mentally comfortable, but, as the years passed, the amount of discomfort which could provoke a nervous disturbance became less and less. She was a well-informed woman, quite interesting on many subjects, outside of herself, and had done much excellent reading. Unafflicted, she would mentally have been more than usually interesting. When her specialist began the investigation of her moral self, he found her impressed with the belief that she was a "saved woman," ready and only waiting health that she might take up the Lord's work. But as he sought her soul's deeper recesses, he uncovered a quagmire. Resentment rankled against the sister who had left her alone to meet the exhausting burdens of their parents' illness and brother's drinking--a sister who had taken care of herself and her own family, regardless. Worse than resentment smoldered against the father, a dull, deadening enmity, born in the hateful hours of his odious, but helpless, dementia. Burning deep was an unappeased protest that, instead of the normal life and pleasures and opportunities of other girls, she had been chained to his objectionable presence.

Treatment was undertaken, based upon a clear conception of her moral, mental and physical needs. Seven months of intensive right-living were enjoined. The greatest difficulty was found in compelling restraint from food excesses. The love for good things to eat was theoretically shelved, but, practically, the forces of desire and habit seemed insurmountable. Her craving for "good eats" now and then discouraged her resolutions and she periodically broke over the rigid hospital regimen. But she was helped in every phase of her living. The skin cleared; a hint of the roses returned;

twenty-five pounds of more than useless weight melted away and weeks passed with no threat of spell or chill. She was renewing her youth. A righteous understanding of the lessons which her years of sacrifice held, appealed to her judgment, if not to her feelings, and, as a new being, she returned to the church training-school.

Most fully had Miss Denny been instructed in principle and in practice concerning the, for her, vital lessons of nutritional right-living. Each step of the way had been made clear, and it had proven the right way by the test of practical demonstration. The outlined schedule of habits, including some denials and some gratuitous activity, kept her in prime condition--in fact, in improving condition, for six highly satisfactory months. Never had she accomplished so much; never did life promise more, as the result of her own efforts. She had earned comforts which had apparently deposed forever her old nervous enemies. Victorious living seemed at her finger-tips. Then she sold her birth- right.

She was feeling so well; why could she not be like other people? Certainly once in a while she could have the things she "loved." It was only a small mess of pottage--some chops, a cup of real coffee, some after-dinner mints. The doctor had proscribed them all, but "Once won't hurt." Her conscience did prick, but days passed; there was no spell, no chill, no headache. "It didn't hurt me" was her triumphant conclusion; and again she ventured and nothing happened--and again, and again. Then the coffee every day and soon sweets and meats, regardless; then coffee to keep her going. The message of the returning fainting spells was unheeded, unless answered by recklessness, for fear thoughts had come and old enmities and new ones haunted in. Routine and regimen had gone weeks before, and now a vacation had to be. She did not return to her work, but deluded herself with a series of pretenses. Before the year was gone, the imps of morbid toxins came into their own and she resorted to wines, later to alcohol in stronger forms--and alcohol usually makes short work of the fineness God gives woman.

We leave Clara Denny at forty, leave her on the road of license which leads to ever-lowering levels.

CHAPTER VII

THE CRIME OF INACTIVITY

A half-century ago the Stoneleighs moved West and located in Hot Springs. The wife had recently fallen heir to a few thousand dollars, which, with unusual foresight, were invested in suburban property. Mr. Stoneleigh was a large man, one generation removed from England, active, and noticeably of a nervous type. He was industrious, practically economical, single-minded; these qualities stood him in the stead of shrewdness. From their small start he became rapidly wealthy as a dealer in real estate. Mr. Stoneleigh was a generous eater; his foods were truly simple in variety but luxurious in their quality and richness. Prime roast-beef, fried potatoes, waffles and griddle-cakes supplied him with heat, energy and avoirdupois. He suddenly quit eating at fifty-eight--there was a cerebral hemorrhage one night. His remains weighed one hundred and ninety-five.

The wife was a comfortable mixture of Irish and English. Her people were so thrifty that she had but a common-school education. She was the only child, her industrious mother let her go the way of least resistance, and were we tracing responsibility of the criminality behind our tragedy, Mrs. Stoneleigh's mother would probably be cited as the guilty one. The way of least resistance is usually pretty easy- going, and keeps within the valley of indulgence. Therefore, Mrs. Stoneleigh worked none, was a true helpmate to her husband, at the table, and like him, grew fat, and from mid-life waddled on, with her hundred and eighty pounds. She was superstitiously very religious, with the kind of religion that shudders at the thought of missing Sunday morning service or failing to be a passive attendant at the regular meetings of the Church Aid Society. Practically, the heathen were taught American civilization, and she herself was assured sumptuous reservations in Glory by generous donations to the various missionary societies.

The only real ordeal which this woman ever faced was the birth of Henry, her first child; she was very ill and suffered severely. The mother instinct centered upon this boy the fulness of her devotion--a devotion which never swerved nor faltered, a devotion which never questioned, a devotion which became a self-forgetting servility. John arrived almost unnoticed three years later, foreordained to be this older brother's henchman as long as he remained at home. John developed. Education was not featured in the Stoneleighs' program, so John stopped after his first year at high school, but he was energetic, and through serving Henry had learned to work. At twenty he married, left the family roof, and starting life for himself in a nearby metropolis became a successful coal-merchant.

Little Henry Stoneleigh would have thrilled any mother's heart with pride. He had every quality a perfect baby should have, and grew into a large handsome boy, healthy and strong; his disposition was the envy of neighboring mothers; nor was it the sweet goodness of inertia, for he was mentally and emotionally quick and responsive above the average. Indulged by his mother from the beginning and always preferred to his brother, he never recognized duty as duty. This young life was innocent of anything which suggested routine; order for him was a happen-so or an of-course result of his mother's or John's efforts; the details necessary for neatness were never allowed to ruffle his ease nor to interfere with his impulses. The Stoneleighs' home was a generous pile, locally magnificent, but our young scion's fine, front room was perennially a clutter. From his birth up, Henry was never taught the rudiments of responsibility. His boyhood, however, was not unattractive. He had inherited a large measure of vitality and was protected from disappointments or irritations by the many comforts which a mother's devotion and wealth can arrange and provide. His memory was superior. The boy inherited not only an exceptional physique, but mental ability which made his early studies too easy to suggest any objection on his part. In fact, he was actively interested in much of his school work and did well without the conscious expenditure of energy. Little discrimination was shown in the arrangements for his higher education; still he arrived at a popular Western Boy's Academy, rather dubious in his own mind as to just how large a place he would hold in the sun, with mother and John back home. Rather rudely assailed were some of his easy-going habits, and considerable ridicule from certain sources rapidly decided his choice of companions. It was young Stoneleigh's misfortune that at this epoch in his development he was situated where money could buy immunities and attract apparent friendships. He was of fine appearance, and should by all rights have made center on the Academy football team, being the largest, heaviest, strongest boy in school. But one day in football togs is the sum of his football history. Academy days went in good feeds, the popularity purchased by his freedom of purse and easy-going good fellowship, and much reading, which he always enjoyed and which, with his good memory, made him unusually well-informed. Finals even at this Academy demanded special effort, which, with Henry, was not forthcoming, so he returned home without his diploma. This incident decided him not to attempt college, so for a year he again basked in the indulgences of home-life. His father's business interests had no appeal for him, but the personal influence of a young doctor, with his vivid tales of medical-college experiences, and the struggling within of a never recognized ambition, with some haphazard suggestions from his mother, determined him to study medicine.

At this time a medical degree could still be obtained in a few schools at the end of two years' attendance. Henry chose a Tennessee college which has, for reasons, long since ceased to exist, an institution which practically guaranteed diplomas. Here after three very comfortable years, he was transformed into "Doc" Stoneleigh. At twenty-five, "Doc" weighed two hundred and forty, and returned home for another period of rest. He did not open an office, nor did he ever begin the practice of his profession. During the next five years he lived at home, sleeping and reading until two in the afternoon, his mother carrying breakfast and lunch to his room. The late afternoons and evenings he spent in hotel-lobbies and pool-rooms, where he was always welcomed by a bunch of sports. Popular through his small prodigalities, he, at thirty, possessed a more than local reputation for the completeness of his assortment of salacious stories--his memory and native social instinct were herein successfully utilized. "Doc" now weighed two hundred and eighty-five, ate much, exercised none, and was the silent proprietor of a pool-room, obnoxious even in this wide-open town.

At twelve he had begun smoking cigarettes; at twenty he smoked them day and night. The entire family drank beer, but, oddly, the desire for alcohol never developed with him. Yet at thirty he began acting queerly, and it was generally thought that he was drinking. Often now he did not go home at night and was frequently found dead asleep on one of his pool-tables. He had fixed up a den of a room where they would move him to "sleep it off." A fad for small rifles developed till he finally had over twenty of different makes in his den and spent many nights wandering around the alleys, shooting rats and stray cats. Eats became an obsession. They invaded his room and he would frequently awaken suddenly and empty the first gun he reached at their imaginary forms, much to the disquiet of the neighbors. One night he burst out of his place, began shooting wildly up and down the street and rushing about in a frenzy. No single guardian of the peace presumed to interfere with his hilarity, and two of the six who came in the patrol-wagon had dismissed action for deep contemplation before he was safely locked up as "drunk." The matter was kept quiet, as befitted the prominence of the Stoneleighs.

To his mother's devotion now was added fear, and she freely responded to his demands for funds. There were no more outbreaks, but he was obviously becoming irresponsible, and influences finally secured his mother's consent to take him to a special institution in another state. This was quietly effected through the cooperation of the family physician, who successfully drugged poor "Doc" into pacific inertness. He was legally committed to an institution empowered to use constructive restraint, and for four months benefited by the only wholesome training his wretched life had ever known. Here it was discovered that he had been using quantities of codein and cocain, against the sale of which there were then no restrictions. Unusual had been his physical equipment, his indulgences unchecked by any sentiment or restraint, the penalty of inactivity was meting a horrible exaction--an exaction which could be dulled only by dope. In the early prime of what should have been manhood, this unfortunate's mind, as revealed to the institution's authorities during his days of enforced drugless discomfort, was a filthy cess-pool; cursings and imprecations, vile and vicious, were vomited forth in answer to every pain. His brother, his doctors, his mother were execrated for days, almost without ceasing. Here was a man without principle. As he became more comfortable, physically, he became more decent, and later his natural, social tendencies began to reappear attractively.

At the end of four months the patient was perforce much better. He then succeeded in inducing his mother to have him released "on probation." Many fair promises were made. For months he was to have an attendant as a companion. His mother, believing him well, consented, after securing his promise in writing to return for treatment should there be a relapse into his old habits. As evidencing the decay of his character, these fair promises were made without the slightest intention that they would be kept. The first important city reached after crossing the state-line saw his demeanor change. Beyond the legal authority of the state in which he had been committed, he was free, and he knew it. With a few words he consigned his now helpless attendant to regions sulphurous, and alone took train in the opposite direction from home. For several months he went the paces. With his medical knowledge and warned by his recent experiences he was able to so adjust his doses as to avoid falling into the hands of the authorities. The weak mother never refused to honor his drafts. Six months later a serious attack of pneumonia caused her to be sent for, and when he was able to travel she took him back to the home he had forsworn.

For over ten years "Doc" Stoneleigh has lived with his mother, a recluse, a morphin-soaked wreck. Sometimes he may be seen in a park near their home, sitting for hours inert, or automatically tracing figures in the gravel with his cane, noticing no one, unkempt, almost repellent. He is still sufficiently shrewd to secure morphin in violation of the law. Sooner or later the revenue department will cut off his supply. He drifts, a rotting hulk of manhood, unconsciously nearing the horrors of a drugless reality.

The depth of this man's degradation may tempt us to feel that he was defective, but an accurate analysis of his life fails to reveal any deficiency save that reprehensible training which made possible his years of physical and mental indolence.

CHAPTER VIII

LEARNING TO EAT

It was three in the early July afternoon. The large parlor, which had been turned into a bedroom, was darkened by closely-drawn shades; a dim, softened light coming from a half-hidden lamp deepened the dark rings around the worn nurse's eyes--eyes which bespoke sleepless nights and a heavy heart. A wan mother stood near the nurse, every line of her face showing the pain of lengthened anxiety. Tensely one hand held the other, the restraint of culture, only, keeping her from wringing them in her anguish. Dr. Harkins, the village physician, stood at the foot of the bed, his honest face set in strong lines in anticipation of the worst. Many scenes of suffering had rendered him only more sympathetic with human sorrow, sympathetic with the real, increasingly intolerant of the false. At the bed-side stood the expert, who had come so far, at so great an expense-long, rough miles by auto that a few hours might be saved-who had come, they all believed, to decide the fate of the beloved girl who lay so death-like before them.

Ruth Rivers was the only one in the room who was not keenly alert or distressingly tense. Even in her waxy whiteness and unnatural emaciation, her face was good. The forehead was high and, with the symmetrical black eyebrows and long, dark lashes, suggested at a glance the good quality of her breeding. The aquiline nose was pinched by suffering, the finely curving lips were now bloodless and drawn tight from time to time, as though to repress the cry of pain; these marks of suffering could not rob her countenance of its refinement. Her breathing was shallow; at times it seemed irregular; and wan, almost inert, the fragile figure seemed nearing the eternal parting with its soul. The silence of the sick-room was fearsomely ominous.

Three weeks before, Ruth, her mother, and ever-apprehensive Aunt Melissa had come from the heat of coastal Georgia to the invigorating coolness of the Southern Appalachians. They had come to Point View several weeks later than usual this year, as spring was tardy and the hot days at home had been few. Ruth had been most miserable for weeks before they left home, but had stood the trip well, and Judge Rivers had received an encouraging, indeed a hopeful report from the invalid. But a few days later a letter telling of another of Ruth's attacks was followed immediately by an urgent, distressed telegram which caused him to adjourn court and hasten to his family.

For many years Dr. Harkins had driven through the mountains eight starving months, serving and saving the poorly housed and often destitute mountaineers. The tourist flood from the burning, summer lowlands to the mountains' refreshment gave him his living. Dr. Harkins was as truly a missionary as though he were on the pay-roll of a denominational society. He had always helped, or the mountains had helped, or something had helped Ruth before, but this time nothing helped. The doctor had already called a neighboring physician; they were both perplexed, and each feared to say the word which, in their minds, spelled her doom. For nearly three days Ruth had been delirious, this gentle, sensible, reserved girl, tossing and calling out. A few times she had even screamed, and her mother always said that she had been "too fine a baby to even cry out loud." For five nights there had been no sleep save an unnatural stupor produced by medicine. Mother and nurse had taxed their strength keeping her in bed during the paroxysms of her suffering, which, hour by hour, seemed to grow in intensity and to defy the ever-increasing doses of quieting drugs. She had recognized no one for days. Even her mother's voice brought back no moment of natural response. "It must be meningitis," Dr. Harkins finally said, and the other doctor nodded in agreement. And Aunt Melissa informed the neighbors that it was "meningitis" and that her darling Ruth could last but a few days. The mother's anxiety reiterated "meningitis," and good, levelheaded Martha King, the nurse, knew that the three cases of meningitis which she had nursed had suffered the same way before they died. When Judge Rivers came, he spent but one minute in the sick-room. It was days before he dared reenter. Ruth did not know him. For the first time in her twenty-seven years, she had failed to respond happily to his hearty, rich-voiced love-greeting. The Judge's small fortune had grown slowly. Only that year had the mortgage been finally lifted on their comfortable Georgia home. But in that minute at the sufferer's bedside all he had was thrown into the scales. Ruth must be saved. She was the only daughter; she was a worthily beloved daughter. "No, she cannot be moved to Johns Hopkins; the trip is too rough and long; she is too weak," decided Dr. Harkins, and the consultant agreed. "Our only hope for her is to get the 'brain expert' from the next state." Five days had passed since the patient had retained food. For twenty-four hours the tide of her strength seemed only to ebb. They all counted the minutes. The summer- boarders in the little town, so many of whom knew the sick girl, counted the hours, for Ruth was much quieter--too quiet, they felt. An hour before, Aunt Melissa had tiptoed in to see her darling; the finger-tips seemed cold in her excited palm, the nails looked bluish to her dreading eyes, and she retreated to the back porch-steps, threw her apron over her head and sat weaving to and fro, inconsolate; nor would she look up even when the big motor panted into sight out of a cloud of dust, and stopped. "It is too late, too late," moaned Aunt Melissa. Dr. Harkins and Judge Rivers met the neurologist. The former reviewed the case in a few sentences. The Judge simply said: "Doctor, my whole savings are nothing. I would give my life for hers."

In the sick-room tensity had given place to intensity, as with deft, skillful directness the doctor made his examination. He had finished; the light had again been dimmed, and in the added shadow the haggard face seemed ashen. Motionless, thoughtful, interminably silent, the expert stood, holding the sick girl's hand. The nurse first saw him smile. It was a serious smile; it was a strangely hopeful smile--a smile which was instantly reflected in her own face and which the mother caught and Dr. Harkins saw. Each one of them was thrilled with such thrills as become rare when the forties have passed, thrilled even before they heard his words: "It is not meningitis. Your daughter can get well."

In the conference which followed, Dr. Harkins felt that his confidence had been well placed. It is surprising how much the expert had discovered in forty minutes,--and how carefully considered and relentlessly logical were his reasons for deciding that it was an "auto-toxic meningismus, secondary to renal and pancreatic insufficiency," which, translated, signifies a self-produced poison due to defective action of the liver and pancreas, resulting in circulatory disturbance in the covering of the brain. Most clearly, too, he revealed that several of the most alarming symptoms were the result of the added poison of the drugs which had been given for the relief of the intolerable pain. Each step of the long road to recovery was outlined with equal clearness, and the light of hope burst in strong on Dr. Harkins first, then on Martha King. The crushing load was lifted from off the Judge's heart. The promise seemed too good to be true, to the mother, who had seen her daughter go down through the years, step by step. It never penetrated the shadow of Aunt Melissa's pessimism.

What forces had been at work to bring ten years of relentlessly increasing suffering, even impending death, to Ruth Rivers at twenty- seven, when she should have been in the glory of her young womanhood? "Her headaches have always been a mystery," her mother had said again and again, and this saying had been accepted by family and friends. Let us join hands with Understanding, step behind this mystery, and find its solution.

Judge Rivers' father had been Judge Rivers, too. The war between the States had absorbed the family wealth; still, our Judge Rivers showed every evidence of good living: he was always well-dressed, as befitted his office, portly and contented, as was also befitting, fine of color and always well. His daughter's illness had been practically the only problem in the affairs of his life which he had not solved to his quite reasonable satisfaction. His love for Ruth held half of his life's sweetness.

Mrs. Rivers was tall, active, almost muscular in type. Her brow, like her daughter's, was high. The quality of her Virginia blood had marked her face. She had always been unduly pale, but never ill. Controlled and reasonable, she had ministered to her home with efficiency and pride.

Aunt Melissa, her sister, five years the senior, was tall and strong, but her paleness had long been unhealthily tinted with sallowness. For years she had been subject to attacks of depression when for days she would insist upon being let alone, even as she let others alone. Ruth was the only bright spot she recognized in her life, and her morbidness was constantly picturing disaster for this object of her love.

Ruth's babyhood was a joy. Plump, cooing and happy, she evinced, even in her earliest days, evidences of her rare disposition. At eighteen months, however, she began having spells of indigestion. She always sat in her high-chair beside Aunt Melissa, at the table, and rarely failed to get at least a taste of anything served which her fancy indicated. Her wise little stomach from time to time expressed its disapproval of such unlawful liberties, but parents and aunts and grandmothers, and probably most of us, are very dull in interpreting the protests of stomachs. So Ruth got what she liked, and what was an equal misfortune, she liked what she got; and no one ever associated the liking and the getting with the poor sick stomach's periodic protests. As a girl Ruth was not very active. There was a certain reserve, even in her playing, quite in keeping with family traditions. Mother, Aunt Melissa and the servants did the work--still Ruth developed, happy, unselfish, kindly and sensitive. There was rigid discipline accompanying certain rules of conduct, and her deportment was carefully molded by the silent forces of family culture. They lived at the county-seat. The public schools which Ruth attended were fairly good. As she grew older, while she remained thin and never approached ruggedness, her digestive "spells" were much less frequent, and during the two years she spent away from home in the Convent, she was quite well, and one year played center on the second basket ball team. Two years away at school were all that the Judge could then afford. And so at eighteen she was home for good. That fall she began having headaches. She was reading much, so she went to Mobile and was carefully fitted with glasses. The correction was not a strong one, but the oculist felt it would relieve the "abnormal sensitiveness of her eyes, which is probably causing her trouble."

Throughout her years of suffering, Ruth had always maintained the rare restraint which marks fineness of soul. No one ever heard her complain. Even her mother could not be sure that another attack was on, until she found Ruth alone in her darkened room. Acquaintances, even friends, never heard her mention her illness.

The midsummer months in Southern Alabama drive such as are able to the relief of the mountains of Tennessee and the Carolinas. The Judge had always felt that he should send his family away during July and August; they often went in June when the summers were early. And these weeks of change proved, year after year, the most helpful influences that came to Ruth. She always improved and would usually remain stronger until after Thanksgiving. But with irregular periodicity the blinding, prostrating headaches would return--a week of pain, nausea and prostration. Yet Ruth never asked for, nor took medicine, unless it was ordered by the doctor, and then more in consideration of the desires of her family, for the unnatural sensations, produced by most of the remedies she was given, seemed but the substitution of one discomfort for another. The only exercise that counted, which this girl ever had, was during her weeks at Point View. The stimulation of the invigorating mountain air seemed to get into her blood, and after a few weeks with her friendly mountains she could climb the highest with little apparent fatigue. At home, the country was flat, the roads sandy, and even horseback riding uninteresting. She had never been taught any strengthening form of daily home-exercise, and so she suffered on. While the glasses brought comfort, they lessened, for but a short time, the number and the intensity of her attacks. Several physicians were consulted and several varying courses of treatment undertaken, but no betterment came which lasted, and the headaches remained a mystery, not only to her mother, but to others who seriously tried to help. As we are behind the scenes, we need no longer delay the mystery's solution. It was not eyes, they were accurately corrected; it was not stomach, as much stomach treatment proved; it was not anaemia, or the many excellent tonics that had been prescribed would have cured; it was not displaced vertebrae nor improperly acting nerves, or the manipulations and vibrations and deep kneadings of the specialists in mechanical treatment would have rescued her years before. It was, and here is the secret--her mother's wonderful table!

The war had brought ruinous, financial losses to most Virginia families. As a result, Ruth's mother had been taught, in minute detail, the high art of the best cookery of the first families of Virginia. And how she could cook, or make the colored cook cook! The Rivers' table had, for years, been the standard of the county-seat. Mrs. Rivers' spiced hams, fig preserves, brandied plum-pudding, stuffed roast-duck, fruit salads, all made by recipes handed down through several generations, could not be excelled in richness and toothsomeness. No simple dishes were known at the Rivers' table; these, for those poor mortals who knew not the inner art. Double cream, stimulating seasonings, sauces rarely spiced, the sort that recreate worn-out appetites, were never lacking at a Rivers' meal. Ruth had been overfed, had been wrongly fed since babyhood.

The expert said hope lay in taking her back to babyhood and feeding her for days as though she were a four months' child. He said she must be taught to eat; that her salvation lay in a few foods of plebeian simplicity, foods which almost any one could get anywhere, foods which did not involve long hours of preparation according to priceless recipes. He said also that certain other foods were vicious, such matter-of-course foods on the Rivers' table, foods which Mrs. Rivers would have felt humiliated to omit from a meal of her ordering, and he insisted that these must be lastingly denied this young woman with prematurely exhausted, digestive glands. The process of her reeducation, succinctly expressed as it was in a few sentences, called for tedious months of care, of denial and of effort. It demanded that which was more than taxing in many details. So for Ruth Rivers long weeks were spent in a hospital-bed. She was fed on the simplest of foods, each feeding measured with the same care as were her few medicines, for now truly her food was medicine, and her chief medicine was food. Massage seemed at last to bring help, for even in bed she gained in strength.

It was several weeks before her mind was entirely clear, but she was soon being taught the science of food; this included an understanding outline of food chemistry, of the processes of digestion, of food values, of the relation of food to work, of the vital importance of muscular activity and the relation of muscle-use to nervous health. Her beloved sweets and her strong coffee, the only friends of her suffering days, were gradually buried even from thought in this accumulation of new and understood truths--most reasonable and sane truths. Forty pounds she gained in twelve weeks. She had never weighed over one hundred and twenty-five. She has never weighed less than one hundred and forty-five since, and, as she is five feet eight, her one hundred and forty-five pounds brought her a new symmetry which, with her high-bred face, transformed the waxen invalid into an attractive beauty. She learned to do manual work. She learned to use every muscle the Lord had given her, every day she lived. An appetite unwhipped by condiments or unstimulated by artifice, an appetite for wholesome food, has made eating a satisfaction she never knew in the old days.

This was ten years ago. Many changes have come in the Rivers' household, the most far-reaching of which is probably the revolution which shook its culinary department from center to circumference. What saved daughter must be good for them all. Father is less portly, more active, less ruddy. Some of the color he lost was found by the mother. Aunt Melissa disappears into her gloom-days but rarely, and has smiling hours unthought in the past. And Ruth has proven that the mystery was adequately solved. She married the kind of man so excellent a woman should have, and went through the trying weeks of her motherhood and has cared for her boy through the demanding months of early childhood without a complication. And all this in the face of Aunt Melissa's reiterated forebodings!

CHAPTER IX

THE MAN WITH THE HOE

In the early years of the eighteenth century, a hardy family lived frugally and simply on a few, fertile Norman acres. Their home was but a hut of stone and clay and thatch. It was surrounded by a carefully attended vineyard and fruit trees which, in the springtime, made the spot most beautiful. On this May day the passerby would have stopped that he might carry away this scene of perfect pastoral charm. The blossoming vines almost hid the house, the blooming trees perfumed the morning breeze, and it all spoke for simple peace and contentment. But at this hour neither peace nor contentment could have been found within. Pierre, the eldest son, was almost fiercely resenting the quiet counsel of his father and the tearful pleadings of his mother. Pierre loved Adrienne, their neighbor's daughter. The two had grown up side by side, each had brought to the other all that their dreams had wished through the years of waiting. Pierre had long worked extra hours and they both had saved and now, nearing thirty, there was enough, and they could marry. But the edict had gone forth that Huguenot marriages would no longer be recognized by the state; that the children of such a union would be without civil standing. So Pierre and Adrienne had decided to leave France, nor did the protests of their elders delay their going. It was a solemn little ceremony, their marriage, a ceremony practically illegal in their land. Rarely are weddings more solemn or bridal trips more sad, for to England they were starting that same day, never to see their dear France again, never to prune or to gather in the little vineyard, never again to look into the faces of their own kin.

It was not a worldly-wise change. Wages in England were very low and there were no vineyards in that chilly land, and Pierre worked and died a plain English farm-hand, blessed only with health, remarkable strength, and a wretched, but happy home. Much of their parents' sturdiness and independence was passed on into the blood of their four children, two boys and two girls, for in 1748, after long saving, they all left England for America, "the promised land," and sailed for New Amsterdam. Husbandmen they were, and for two generations painfully, gravely, they tilled the semi-productive soil of their little farm, west of the Hudson. Land was cheap in the New World. Their vegetables and fruit grew, the market in the city grew, and the van der Veere farms grew, and peace and contentment abode there.

After the War of 1812 two healthy, robust van der Veere brothers tramped into New York City each carrying in his bundle nearly $1000.00, his share of their father's recently divided farm. They started a green-grocery shop. One attended the customers, the other, through the summer months, worked their little truck garden away out on the country road, a road which is to-day New York's Great White Way. They prospered. One married, and his two boys founded the van der Veere firm of importers. From the East this company's ship, later its ships, brought rare curios, oriental tapestries and fine rugs to make elegant the brown-stone front drawing-rooms of aristocratic, residential New York of that generation. The sons of one of these brothers to-day constitute the honorable van der Veere firm. The other brother left one son, Clifford, and two daughters, Dora and Henrietta. It is into the life-history of Clifford van der Veere that we now intrude. He was a sturdy youth, with no illnesses, save occasional sore throats which left him when he shed his tonsils. His father was a reserved, kindly man, a quietly efficient man. His competitors never understood the sure growth of his success--he was so unpretentious in all that he did. Clifford's mother was a sensible woman, untouched by the pride of wealth and the snobbery of station. Their home, facing Central Park, stood for elegance and restraint. There were no other children for ten years after the son's birth, then came the two sisters, which domestic arrangement probably proved an important factor in deciding the rest of our story. From early boyhood Clifford was orderly, obedient, studious and quietly industrious. He made no trouble for parents or teachers--other mothers always spoke of him as "good." He was thirteen when his only sinful escapade happened. Some of the Third Avenue boys shared the playgrounds in the park with Clifford's crowd. They all smoked, some chewed and the more self- important of them swore, and thereby, one day, our Fifth Avenue young hopeful was contaminated. It was a savory-smelling wad of fine-cut. It burned, a little went the wrong way and it strangled, but the joy of ejecting a series of amber projectiles was Clifford's. Another mouthful was ready for exhibition purposes when some appreciative admirer enthusiastically clapped our boy between the shoulder-blades and most of his mouth's contents, fluid and solid, was swallowed. Somehow Clifford got home, but landed in a wilted heap on the big couch, chalk-white, and sick beyond expression. The doctor was called and, discovering the cause, made him helpfully sicker. The next morning Clifford's father gravely offered to give him $500.00, when he was twenty-one, if he would not taste tobacco again until that time. Either the memory of first-chew sensations or the doctor's ipecac, or the force of habit, or something, kept him from ever tasting it again.

Later, Clifford went to Columbia and was quietly popular with the quieter fellows. It would seem that had any little devils not been strained out of his blood by his long line of Huguenot ancestry, they had followed the fate of the fine-cut, for no one who knew Clifford van der Veere was ever anxious about the probity of his conduct. He did not take to the importing business, while his cousins early showed a natural capacity for the work of the big firm in all its branches. Clifford's parents, too, seemed to feel that it was time that there be a professional member of their honorable family. Moreover the property was large, and the younger sisters would require a guardian, and the estate an administrator. So Clifford finished the law-course. Nor was it many years until the family fortune of approximately one million dollars in real estate, securities and mortgages was left him to administer for himself and the two sisters. Thus before thirty the responsibility of these many thousands swept down upon him. Limited in practical contact with the world, geographically, politically, socially, having learned little of the play-side of life, he was by inheritance, training and inclination a conservative. He had never practiced law. He never tried a case, but he now opened a downtown office where he punctually arrived at ten o'clock and methodically spent the morning, carefully, personally managing all the details of the entailed estate. He was essentially conscientious and, as the years passed, there was no lessening of interest in his devotion to each transaction, large or small. There were no losses, though his conservatism turned him away from many golden opportunities which knocked at the door of his wealth, the acceptance of which would have doubled the estate in any ten-year period of these days of New York's magnificent expansion. He was nearly forty when he married a quiet, good woman who added little that was new, who most conscientiously subtracted nothing of the old, from his now systematic life. They both realized that their Fifth Avenue home was rapidly growing out of date, so for nearly five years they spent their spare hours daily, in the, to Clifford, vital and seemingly unending details of modernizing the old house. It was during those days when the plans so carefully considered were being realized in granite and marble and polished woods, that Mrs. van der Veere felt the first distressing touch of anxiety. Her husband seemed unduly particular. At times he would be painfully uncertain about minute and minor details of construction and on a few occasions unprecedentedly failed to get to the office at all, delayed by protracted discussions of the advisability of certain changes, long since decided upon, discussions which shook the confidence of architect and contractor in both his sagacity and judgment. Fortunately Mrs. van der Veere proved a wholesome counselor and her opinions often settled details her husband, alone, apparently could not have decided. At last the great new house was finished; it was such a home as the van der Veeres should have. Indecision largely disappeared for three quite normal years, office details only now and then ruffling the smooth normality of Mr. van der Veere's life. Then with the early spring nights came an unexplained insomnia. He would waken at five, four, even three o 'clock, and, unable to get back to sleep, would read until morning. The doctor found little to excite his apprehension, but prescribed golf, so three afternoons a week all summer and fall two hours were reserved for the links. He was better, still the doctor insisted on three months, that winter, in Southern California where he could keep up his play. Here he did eighteen holes a day for weeks at a time, yet some of the nights were haunted by scruples about neglecting his administrative duties. They returned home in the spring, and a moderately comfortable year and a half followed. Then things went wrong rapidly and badly. Peremptorily he was ordered away from all "work" to Southern France, later to Italy for the winter and to Switzerland for the next summer. And as the Alps have given of their strength to other needing thousands, so they ministered to him. He began climbing. His wife thought it was a new interest. Certainly that was a factor, but he became ambitious and went wherever he could find guides to take him. He returned home very rugged the fall he was fifty. Still with reason, Mrs. van der Veere was anxious, an anxiety shared by the family doctor. Between them they planned for him a sort of model life, truly a circumscribed life, and for five years wife and associates protected him from any possible strain, and for five years it worked successfully. Then in less than a month, almost like a bolt from the blue, all former symptoms returned, aggravated in form, bringing most unwelcome new ones in their trail. The family doctor called in a neurologist who, after examining the nervous man, spoke seriously of serious possibilities, and advised serious measures.

Mr. van der Veere was now fifty-five years old, short, almost stocky in build, dark-skinned, with steel-gray hair and mustache. He was depressed in mien though always well-bred in bearing. He was not excitable and outwardly showed little of his suffering. Clifford van der Veere had always taken life and his duties seriously. For years his fear of making mistakes had been a chronic source of energy leakage-now it was a nightmare. All he did cost an exhausting price in the effort of decision. Duty and fear had long made a battle-ground of his soul, and when he realized that he had broken down again from "overwork," as they all expressed it, the depression of melancholy was added to the weight he so quietly bore. Yet this man of many responsibilities and interests had never truly worked. Since he left college he had played at work. Effort had been expended never more conscientiously. He was ever ready to give added hours of attention to problems referred to him. His intentions were true, but he did not know how to work. He did not know how to separate the serious from the unimportant, and he had never added the leaven of humor to the day's duties. An unusually well-equipped man, physically and mentally, he should have found the responsibilities of his administratorship but play. Had he been living right, he could have multiplied his efficiency three-fold and been the better for the larger doing. His wife felt he must "rest," and so did the family doctor; he himself was practically past arguing or disagreeing.

But the rest-cure which the neurologist prescribed was certainly unique. It may have been wrongly named. Mr. van der Veere was a man of unusually strong physique. Nature had equipped him with a muscular system better than nine-tenths of his fellowmen possess, but he had never utilized it. For many generations his forbears had wrung food and life and, unconsciously, health from the soil. He was three generations from touch with mother earth, and back to the soil he was sent. He was taught to work increasing hours of common, manual labor. For weeks he did his part of the necessary drudgery of the world. He shoveled coal, he spaded in the garden, he worked on the public roads, he transplanted trees, he hoed common weeds with a common hoe, he tramped, he toiled and he sweat. The need for physical labor was in his blood. He needed his share of it, as do we all. And his blood answered exultantly, as good blood always does, to the call of honest toil. Within a month he realized a keenness for the work of the day. His fine muscles took on hardness, they seemed to double in size, and strength came, and with it not only a willingness but an eagerness which transformed that strength into productive effort. With the willingness to do what his hands found to do came sleep, for his nerves--bred as they had been in good stock--rejoiced when they found him living as they had for years begged him to live. A fifteen-year- old appetite came to the fifty-five-year-old man, and transformation wrought happy changes in his face and bearing. Indecision faded, introspection disappeared, and a decision came which was to forever put indecision out of his way. A decision which brought the peace and contentment to the van der Veere Fifth Avenue home, which religious intolerance had robbed from the van der Veeres in their stone-thatched hut in far-away Normandy, a simple decision, not requiring brilliance nor a college education, nor a professional training, nor even a loving helpmate to accomplish: "Six days shall I labor not only with my brain but with my hands, and the seventh day shall I rest."

CHAPTER X

THE FINE ART OF PLAY

It was her earliest recollection, and parts of it were not clear. There were those big men carrying in her father, and her mother's face looking so strange, and her father looking so strange with the white cloths about his head, and the strange faces of doctors and neighbors she had not seen before. Then the strange stillness and the strange new fear when her father did not move and they all were so quiet. These memories were rather blurred; she was not always sure which were memories of the events or which had grown from what she had afterwards heard. But of the funeral she was very sure, for she could never forget those beautiful silvered handles on the shining wooden coffin, or her resentment toward the women dressed in black who would not let her touch these--the prettiest things she had ever seen. The colts had run away, frightened, when an empty sap-barrel fell off the sled, and her father had been thrown against a tree and brought home with a fractured skull, to live unconscious two days, and to be buried in the shiny coffin with the silver handles.

There had been an older child who died as a baby of eight months, and so Widow Gilmore was left at thirty-five with her only child, Hattie, and a hundred-and-forty-acre farm, with the house in town. Mrs. Gilmore had good business sense. She lived alone with Hattie, ran the farm, and soon her interests degenerated into a slavery to household and farm details.

The widow had taught school until she was nearly thirty. She was not handsome, and the meager sentiment of her soul easily disintegrated into morbidness. She wore black the rest of her days, and for the rest of her days church services were hours of public mourning. The Gilmore "parlor" was closed after the funeral, and Hattie never got a glimpse within its almost gruesomely sacred walls, save as she timidly peeped in during cleaning days or, rarely, when her mother tearfully led her in and they stood before the life-size crayon portrait of the departed. Even in her quiet play, Hattie must keep on the other side of the house.

Hattie Gilmore was a sober child and lived a sober childhood. She was not strong; nothing had ever been done to make her so. Play and playmates were always limited. She and her mother belonged to Coopersville's "better class," most of the town children living below the bridge where the homes of the factory people crowded. Boys were "too rough," and the other girls were "not nice enough"; so she played much alone--such play as it was, with her two china dolls and the tin stove and tin dishes, which made up her toys. There was little to stimulate her imagination and nothing to develop comradeships and friendships. For hours of her play-time she sat inertly on the front stoop and watched the passersby, for there had never been any thought of training her in the art of play. Instead, she was warned to keep her dress clean and rather sharply reprimanded if, perchance, dress or apron was torn. So she stood and watched the school-play of the other children, never knowing the thrills of a game of "tag," nor the reckless adventures of "black man"; even

"Pussy wants a corner" disarranged her painfully curled curls and was rarely risked. "Hop- scotch," when the figure was small and lady-like, was practically the limit of Hattie's "violent exercise." So she did not develop-how could she! She remained undersized. Moreover, her play-days were sadly shortened, for they early merged into work-days. Housekeeping cares were many, as her mother planned her household. According to York State traditions Hattie was early taught domestic details, and for over a generation seriously, slavishly followed the routine established by her mother who doggedly, to the last, knew no shadow of turning, and went to her honestly earned long rest within a week after she took to her bed. Hattie finished the town high school, and had taken her school-work so seriously that she was valedictorian--being too good to soil your dress ought to bring some reward. Her teacher proudly referred to her as an example of the fine work a student could do who was not disturbed by outside influences. Commencement night, the same summer she was seventeen, she was almost pretty. The natural flush of success and of public recognition was heightened by the reflected flush from the red roses she wore; and Ben Stimson, the old doctor's son, carried the image of this, her most beautiful self, in his big heart for many years. He was then twenty, a sophomore at college, and a wholesome fellow to look upon. He took Hattie home that night. It was early June, and they dallied on the way. She was so nearly happy that her conscience became suspicious. She felt something awful was going to happen!--and she almost did not care. They had reached the front steps of her home. Ominously, silence fell. Suddenly impulsive Ben crushed her to him and--must it be told?--kissed her, kissed Hattie Gilmore's unsullied lips. For a moment her heart leaped almost into wanton expression. A moment more--another kiss, and she might have been compromised, she might have responded to the thrilling love which was calling to her heart, but the goddess of her destiny willed otherwise. The front door opened; an angular form appeared; an acrid voice fairly curdled love-thoughts as it assailed the impetuous lover. Within a minute he was slinking away and the rescued maiden was safe in the indignant, resenting arms of her mother--safe, but for years to be tempted and troubled by remorse and wishes, to be haunted by unaccepted hopes. "Ben Stimson is a free lance. He can't help being, for his father's a free thinker and the boy never went to Sunday-school a dozen times in his life. Let him join the church and show folks he wants to live right; then, if he courts you regular, I won't mind, but he is too free and easy. I call that kind dangerous," her mother said.

Ben Stimson wrote Hattie a note the next day, which she did not answer, but kept for years. Two summers later he drove up to the house, looking mighty fine in the doctor's new runabout, driving the high-stepping bay, natty in a "brand-new" tan harness--the first Hattie had ever seen. He asked her to come with him for a drive, and again her mother's nipping negative influenced her decision against the pleadings of a yearning, lonely heart.

Mrs. Gilmore finally died an exclusive, matter-of-fact, joyless death, even as she had lived. Ben came to the funeral. He called on Hattie the next day. Inconstancy was not one of his weaknesses, and the veil of her Commencement beauty had clung to her through these many years, in her old lover's eyes. He was again impetuous and offended every conservative propriety of Hattie's dutiful melancholy by asking her to marry him--and this actually in the room where her mother's funeral was held the day before! What could Hattie do but burst into tears and leave the room--and Ben, and the secretly cherished hopes of many years, and a real home with a cheerily happy husband and those children which might have been hers--to leave all these and more in homage to the sacredness of her mother's memory.

Ten gray years dragged by. Hattie kept a few boarders so as not to be alone in the house. She would take no children. They were too noisy and kept the place in disorder. Ben's patience had finally exhausted, though he finished his medical course and had been practicing nearly ten years before he married. No other one for whom she could care even called.

The farm did well. The lone woman had over $20,000 in the bank and the property was worth as much more. But the brightest days were gray. At forty-five she weighed ninety-four. She ate barely enough to keep going. Her digestion was wretched. Her pride and her will alone made her able to sit through meals or through the occasional neighbors' calls. She spent hours alone in her room, dumb, dark-minded, with an unrelenting heartache and pains which racked every organ. Her sleep was fitful and she dreamed of Ben downstairs in a casket, again and again, until she fairly feared the night. When she took her nerve medicine, she seemed tied, bound hand and foot in that parlor of death, held by a sleep of terror. Then Ben would move about in the casket and make tortured faces at her, and some horrible times he accused, even berated her. Finally an awful dream, two caskets, her mother in one, Ben in the other, each railing and both showering abuse upon her. She was in bed for weeks. Another doctor came and then- praise be! her deliverer.

Jane Andrews was the old Presbyterian minister's daughter. She had lived in Coopersville until she was twenty-four, giving her father an efficient, devoted daughter's care through his long, last illness. The family means had always been limited, and when the earner was laid away, she at once responded to the practical call. There were no hospitals near; so she left home and went into training in a small institution on the Hudson. This is a hospital where sickness is recognized as more than infections and broken, mangled members. Here she learned well the saving balm of joy in making whole wretched bodies with their more wretched souls. For five years she had lived in the midst of benefits brought by the inspiration of right-feeling attitudes. She knew full well the healing potency of the play-spirit. Her insight into life was already deep, her outlook upon life high and heartful. Then her mother failed; she came home and for three months had been beautifying the final weeks, This more than wise woman now came to nurse poor Hattie, came to companion her back to health, came as a revelation to this mistaken and wearied one, of a better way. After forty-five years of the playless life of a serf to blighting seriousness, the wonder is that sourness had not entered to hopelessly curdle all chances for joyous living.

Hattie Gilmore had to be taught to play. During the weeks of her rest-treatment the stronger woman took the weaker back to girlhood. She brought some dolls. They made clothes for them. They dressed and undressed them and put them to bed. They taught them to say their prayers and prepared their little meals, teaching them "table manners," and they made them play as children should play. A sunshine scrapbook was made. It was a gorgeous conglomeration of colors, of fairies and children, of birds and flowers, and of awkward, but telling, hand-illustrations of the joys of being nursed and, prophetically, of the greater joys of being well. They played "Authors," "Flinch," and even "Old Maid." Splendid half-hours were spent in reading gloriously happy lives. Stories were told--happiness stories, and jokes and conundrums invented. One day Hattie laughed aloud, for which heartlessness her morbid conscience at once wrung forth a stream of tears; but that wondrously artful nurse held a mirror before a woefully twisting face, and her tactful comments brought back the smiles. That laugh was the first warming beam of a summer of happiness which was to golden the autumn of a bleak life made blest. Then Hattie Gilmore learned to play a score of out-of-door games and to understand sports. She learned to see the beauties in the roadside flowers-"weeds" her mother had called most of them. She learned to read glorious stories in the ever-transforming clouds. The neighbors' children were invited, timidly they came at first, later they were eager to come and play at "Aunt Hattie's." Three fine, determining events happened that fall to complete the salvation of this woman who was so fast learning happiness-living.

They, Jane and Hattie, friends now rather than nurse and patient, made the daintiest possible cap and cloak for Dr. Ben's last baby, and sent it with a hearty, merry greeting. This was a peace-offering to the past, more efficient probably than much blood which has been shed on sacrificial altars. Then they made a trip which came near being a solemn occasion, it was so portentously important. They went to the church-orphanage, remained several days and brought home a lusty three-year-old bunch of mischief, who was forever to wreck all the gloom-sanctity of that old home. Hereafter even the parlor of mourning was to be assailed with shouts of glee; some things planted in Hattie's flower beds were foredoomed not to come up; no longer could the front lawn look like a freshly swept carpet. Roy was legally adopted by Hattie and became her proudest possession. Finally, her eyes were opened to that rarely sighted, fair vista of the sacred play-life, the play-life so long denied this good woman. Never again were housekeeping worries to be mentioned. They were not recognized. When things went wrong, they went merrily wrong. What could not be cured was joked about. The whole business of home-making became a gladsome game.

Life for Hattie Gilmore, for Roy, for the neighbors' children, and for some of the mothers of dull old Coopersville came to be lived as the Father intended His children to live, when one almost old woman found the Fountain of Youth revealed by the fine art of play. A blessed revelation it is to every life when the joy of play robs the working hours of their tedium and weariness. He lives as master who makes play of his work.

CHAPTER XI

THE TANGLED SKEIN

Warm balls of comfort, a thousand sheep feed on the hillside, turning herb and green growing things into food and wool. After the shearing and the washing, ten thousand soft strands are spun into a single thread, and each length of thread is a promise of warmth and protection for years to come. Then the wool-white yarn is dyed in colors symbolizing the strength of the navy, the loyalty of the army or the honor of the alma mater. Reeled into a skein, the wool is now all but ready for the fingers of the knitter; it has but to be wound in a ball. Yet here danger lurks. An inadvertent twist or a simple tangle quickly knots the thread, unless thoughtful patience rescues. Recklessness means hopeless disarray, and the soft fluff of warming color becomes unkempt disorder, a confused mass from which the thread broken again and again is extracted. The work of careful hands has been reduced to lasting defect.

Francis Weston was reared in one of the prosperous, middle-Western cities, on the northern bank of the Ohio. The family had succeeded well and represented large manufacturing interests. All burdens which money could lift were removed, from his shoulders. He finished college in the East and entered business, never having felt a hand's weight of responsibility. As vice-president and director in one of the banks organized largely by the family's capital, he was free to follow his impulses. No details demanded his attention; other minds in the bank cared for these.

Across the river a southern town nestled in cozy comfort, having for generations maintained a conscious superiority to its smoking, northern neighbor. Several handsome daughters of Kentucky aristocracy gave tangible evidence of the tone of the community, and Francis Weston's impulses made his trips across the river increasingly frequent. And, as it should have been, North and South were joined closer by one more golden link, when an only daughter of Kentucky wealth became Mrs. Weston. The marriage contract held but one stipulation: their home was to be in the bride's village. It looked as though one of Love's best plans had succeeded. The husband proved deeply devoted to his wife and the new home. The bank continued to take most excellent care of itself, and his trips north, across the river, were but occasional. The Weston mansion and estate in every way befitted the combined wealth of the two families, and the wife gave much time to making it increasingly attractive, and to the training of her good servants. The husband read much, exercised little, and the only reason for gentle protest from the wife was his excessive smoking.

A little daughter came, but as though Fate would say, "I am Master," she lived but a few days. The shock was cruel, and the father seemed to suffer the more intensely. Mrs. Weston took her sorrow in a fine way; she seemed to realize that she, of the two, must turn away the threat of morbidness. But the touch of Fate was not to be denied. Still, three years later, it would seem that nothing but thankfulness and abounding joy should have filled the Weston home--a son came. They named him Harold. The father's solicitude for the little fellow's life was as pathetic as it was abnormal. The bank was now unvisited for months by its first vice-president. As the boy grew the father gave him more and more of himself. He was his companion in play, and personally taught him, seriously taking up study after study, until at sixteen Harold was well prepared for college--scholastically prepared, we should amend--for unconsciously the father had kept him from the normal comradeship with boys of his age. Much of excellent theory the youth had, some wisdom beyond his years, but no knowledge of denials, no spirit of give and take, no thought of the other fellow--his rights and wrongs. In spite of their long walks and rides on gaited Kentucky thoroughbreds, Harold was not physically robust, so it was decided to send him to a southern college, and he went to Vanderbilt. During his second year the father had a long siege of typhoid, and recovery was pitiably imperfect. His mentality did not return with his body strength--he remained a harmless, weak-minded man. Much care was exercised to keep the details from Harold, though both families were unwilling to have the broken man sent to an institution, and for four years professional nurses attended him at home. In spite of the mother's best efforts to distract and neutralize, the son could but feel the unnaturalness of the home atmosphere and profoundly miss the devotion of his father. Still from what little he did see of the invalid, it was a relief when, four years later, an accident took him away.

Harold Weston's college life held true to his training. Quietly friendly, he mixed poorly; mentally well-equipped, he was an excellent student--brilliant in some classes, good in all. Athletics and fraternities, feeds and "femmies" dissipated none of his energies, nor added aught to the fulness of his living. He continued his college work until he had received both Bachelor's and Master's degrees. The spring he was twenty-three, he returned home for the summer, an attractive young man. A classmate had interested him in tennis, for which he showed some natural aptitude. The year's work had taxed him lightly. The skein of yarn gave promise of a perfect fabric.

Mother and son had a happy summer. She saw to it that the home was alive with young folks, and one week-end party followed another. Harold had decided to study law, and nothing indicated that he would meet any obstacles during his course at Law School. All believed he was sufficiently strong to take this at Yale. There were brilliant minds in his classes--he was accustomed to lead. He dropped his tennis, he studied hard. In his second year he began losing weight after the holidays, and found difficulty in getting to sleep; his appetite became irregular, and his smoking, which had been moderate for some years, became a dependence. His nervous system was pretty well "shot up"--it had never been case-hardened. A weight of apprehension had become constantly present, and he let its burden depress him miserably. One of his professors, noting his appearance, talked with him earnestly, and with lay acumen decided his digestion was "out of fix" and told him of a "fine New York doctor." The stomach specialist worthily stood high in his profession. The examination was painstaking and exhaustive; the diagnosis seemed ominous to the morbid patient; the whole process was a revelation to him of organs and functions and laws of eating and drinking unheard in his years of study. "Chronic intestinal indigestion with food decomposition and auto-intoxication, augmented by nicotine," the doctor said. There had been a distinct lessening of efficiency in his law-school work. Study for the first time in his life required wearying effort. He did not feel himself, he was facing his first test, he was meeting his first strain. For the first time the skein was being mussed.

Harold Weston began reading, indiscriminately, literature on food and digestion and diets. The doctor had given him a strict regimen. He began to note minutely the foods he ordered and to question the wholesomeness of their quality and preparation. Caution and over emphasis on details of food and habits of eating rapidly developed. Later not only the food in the dish, but most unhappily the foods he had swallowed were scrutinized by every alertness of sensation and imagination, and most damagingly did he become a victim of the unwholesome symptom-studying habit. Within two months his discerning physician recognized that the self-interest which had started in the physical damage of rapid eating of rich foods was developing into an obsession more detrimental than the original physical disorder, and thought it wise for him to discontinue study and return home to rest for the summer.

The thread was tangled.

The home-coming was not happy. From the first meal, the specialist's warnings were in conflict with the home diet, and resentments were not withheld from the good old dishes which had for a generation bedecked the home table. The delicacy instinctive to the family and to his earlier life was cast aside, and the subjects of food and its digestion, of food-poisoning and its consequences, made unpleasant every meal. Innocently and seriously the mother pointed to her good health and to rugged ancestors who had lived long and hale, unconsciously superior to food and drink. He brooked none of her suggestions, and finally when she honestly could not see it all his way, in the heat of his intensity he accused her of being to blame for all his trouble: she had fed him wrong from the first; she had fed his father wrong; the New York doctor had told him that certain mental diseases could be caused by food-poisoning, and his father would not have been a mental wreck, nor his own career cut short, had she only known what wives and mothers of this generation should know, and set a table which was not a laboratory of poison. These ideas, once accepted, never left him. They formed a theme which, after finding expression, recurred with ominously increasing frequency. A year before, Harold Weston was a kindly fellow, almost retiring, but with a peculiar lighting of his face in response which endeared him to feminine hearts. On a variety of subjects he was well-informed, his professors bespoke for him a high and honorable standing in the judiciary, but, from the mass of this fine mind's possibilities, a second wretched choice was now made. "Father's typhoid affected his mind, his brain must have been defective; my heredity is imperfect; my first illness damages my class work. I can never go on in my profession, there is no future for me but suffering." From this wrecking thought it was an easy step to condemnation of his father for his fatherhood, which, with his near-enmity toward his mother for her "criminal ignorance" in rearing him, introduced a sordidly demoralizing element into his mind which forever viciously tinctured memories and relations which should have been his sacred helpers. The normal mind can select well its world--miserably his mind lived with these dregs of his own choice. The power of normal selection will, in the best mind, be gradually lost through habitual surrender to the morbid.

For the next year he lived unhappily in a home which he made unhappy. Naturally thoughtful, he daily took long walks, brooding over his wrongs--

walks which brought him little benefit physically, as he considered himself unable to put into them sufficient effort to wring perspiration from his brow or toxins from his muscles. False interpretation of his own symptoms increased with the abnormal closeness of his scrutiny of them. His superficial knowledge he accepted as final. Ignorant of the limitations of heredity, will and judgment became subservient to pessimism, and the days marked a gradual, deepening depression. The skein was asnarl.

A relative physician responded to the mother's call of distress and spent a week in the home, then took Harold under his personal care to a series of specialists--but not stomach specialists. Serious treatment was carried out at home with a young physician as companion. Two institutions offered the best help of their elaborate equipments and perfected methods. Three years of badly discounted usefulness passed. Long since had any call of responsibility ceased to elicit response. Toward the end of this time he seemed better, and was spending the summer at a health-resort, living a relatively normal life. Fate then seemed to smile--dainty fingers appeared from the nowhere, which promised gently, patiently, surely to loosen each tangled snarl.

Eva Worth was another only child of affluence. She, too, was recuperating, spending the summer at the same resort as Harold. "Overwork at college," it was said. Petite of person, pleasing in manner, sweetly spoiled, with sympathies quickly born but usually displaced by fresher interests, she was bright and responsive in mind, and her attraction to Harold Weston gave promise of being the touch needed to complete his restoration. Providence only knows the possibilities latent in a union of these poor children of wealth. For him there was an unquestioned awakening. The somber clouds of his moods seemed destined to be transformed into delicate pastels by the promises of love. It was more than an infatuation for them both, and an understanding which was virtually an engagement left them happy even in their parting. But happiness was not a word for Harold Weston's conjuring. Throughout the weeks of his association with this fair girl, the first woman for whom he had ever cared, the thought had repeatedly come that he owed her a full and explicit explanation of his illness and of his "defective heredity." At home where the brooding habit had grown strong and fixed, this idea became so insistent, within two weeks, that he relieved the tension of its demands by a long letter of details, which even to the sympathetic ear of love were more than disquieting. The letter ended with a question of her willingness to indicate a final decision in her response. The appeal of his fine eyes was not there to help--other eyes were nearer. Eva Worth was but twenty-two. Home training, the reading of much fine literature, a college education, her own poor little heart, all failed to bespeak for her wisdom in this crisis. An impulsive, almost resentful refusal was sent. Second thoughts held more wisdom, for woman's pity was now wisdom, so another day saw another letter, one with a few saving words of hope. The first reply was handed to Harold after luncheon. Quietly he left the house, apparently for one of his afternoon walks. By morning he had not returned and a general alarm went out. Some days later two boys, fishing in the river from an old log, saw a cap in an eddy. No more has been seen or heard of Harold Weston. A hasty hand, a hasty touch had broken the thread.

Two women were left to suffer. The elder, haunted by the re-echoings of an only son's condemnation, lives out her years in a loneliness which will not break, harrowed by questions of the wisdom of her mother-love, the best she had to give. Some mother's son she may yet help save, for she knows the vital error which shielded and guarded her boy till he reached his majority, never having met trial, hopelessly untrained in coping with adversity. The younger, sobered by the voice of self-accusation, ever feels the weight of the consciousness of a grave duty slighted; she was made more wise in a day of deep reality than by twenty years of conventional training. Tested again she would give as she has never known giving, give that she might protect.

CHAPTER XII

THE TROUBLED SEA

A young woman, of rather striking appearance attired in her street clothing, is standing beside her dresser. She has just returned from town. She is of medium height, trim of figure, weighing about one hundred and forty, with skin of a soft ivory tint and cheeks showing a faint flush of health--or of excitement. Her dark hair waves gracefully and the scattering strands of gray quite belie her youth. The eyes are well placed, nearly black, and can sparkle on occasion. Her rather poorly formed hands of many restless habits, are the only apparent defect in this, externally attractive, young woman. She has just broken the seal of a heavy vellum envelope addressed in a strange feminine hand. It is an engraved announcement which reads:

"Mrs. Pinkney Rogers announces the marriage of her daughter, Pearl May, to Mr. Lee Burnham"--

She never read the rest. She never saw the--"on Tuesday, May thirtieth nineteen hundred and one. At Home, Rome, Georgia, after July fifth." Her sister, Addie, coming up the stairs, thought she heard a moan and hurried in to find Stella lying in a crumpled heap. Addie's quick eye noticed the announcement. She read it all, and destroyed it, and through the years it was never mentioned by either of them. She, alone, knew its relation to her sister's collapse, but with proverbial southern pride never voiced her opinion of the tragic cause of her older sister's years of nervous ill-health.

Mr. Beckman, Stella's father, was at this time about fifty-five. He was the brunette parent from whom many of her more attractive physical qualities had been inherited. He was proprietor of the best men's furnishing store of the county's metropolis. His business was moderately successful, built up, he felt, entirely through years of his personal thought and attention, and it was practically his only interest. Even his interesting family was a matter of course--though the amount of the day's sales never became so. Mr. Beckman had a single diversion. The store closed at ten o'clock Saturday nights; between twelve and one its proprietor would reach home in an exalted state, and for two hours poor Mrs. Beckman would hear his plans for developing the biggest gent's clothing-business in the state, for becoming a merchant-prince, emphasized with many a hearty slap on her back. This weekly relaxation was always followed by a miserable Sunday morning, invariably referred to by every member of the family as "another of Papa's sick headaches." Mrs. Beckman never lisped the details of those unhappy Saturday nights, and the loyal deception was so well carried out, with such devoted attention and nursing, that by early afternoon, Sunday, the invalid was quite restored and any possible self-reproach had been melted away. Headaches of the real kind did come later, and, as his habits changed not, the Brights which first appeared at fifty-eight progressed without interruption to his death at sixty.

Mrs. Beckman was a blonde, but for many years had been a badly faded one. She was as singleminded in regard to her household as her husband to his store. Neither had developed more than family and local interests. She was the same age as her husband and had, without question, worked faithfully, long hours, through the long years, in homage to her sense of housekeeping duties. The coming of the children, only, from time to time, kept her away from kitchen and parlor for a few weeks. She had been to Atlanta but once during the last ten years, not that Mr. Beckman willed it so--she could have had vacations and attractive dresses, though for some reason, possibly the "fading" which has been mentioned, he never urged her to go with him-- and she needed urging, for she honestly believed there was "too much to do" at home. The habit of industry can become as inveterate as habits of pleasure.

The two Beckman boys had the virtues of both father and mother. They finished at the city high school, and at once went to work in the store with such earnestness of purpose that they were quite prepared to conduct the business, even better than the father had done, when he became incapacitated.

We met the sister, Addie, in Stella's room and realized from her discretion, manifested under stress, that she possessed elements of character. She was a clear-skinned, high-strung blonde--thin-skinned too, probably, for from childhood her hands rebelled at household duties. The family thrift was hers, however, and from the limited opportunities of the home town, she prepared herself for, and filled well, for years, a position with a successful law firm. She later married the senior member--a widower. His children and her high-strung thin-skinnedness and lack of domestic propensities have not made her as successful a home-builder as she was a stenographer.

Stella Beckman's early life was deeply influenced by many of the surroundings which we have glimpsed. Hers was not a home of fine ideals. Much that was common was always present. The table-talk was almost competitive in nature, as, with the possible exception of the mother, each one used "I" almost insistently, as a text for converse, the three times a day they sat together. Even mutual interests were largely obscured, much of the time, by personal ones, barring only the subject of sickness. All forms of illness were themes commanding instant and absorbing attention. Inordinate anxiety was felt by all for the ills of the one; and for days the "I" would be forgotten if any member of the home-circle was "sick." And the concerns of the patient, whether suffering from a cold, sore eyes, a sprained ankle, or "had her tonsils out," were discussed with minuteness of detail worthy an

International Conference. How the patient slept, what the doctor said, the effect of the new medicine, how the heart was standing the strain, what the visiting neighbors thought of the case, in fact the whole subject of sickness held a morbid interest for each member of the family. Sickness, no matter how slight, was with the Beckmans ever an excuse for changing any or all plans. We might speak of the discussion of illness as the Beckman family avocation.

Stella was a bright child, who, wisely directed and influenced, would have taken a good education. She could have developed into a particularly pleasing, capable, useful, possibly forceful woman. But the emotional Stella was over-developed, until it obstructed the growth of the reasoning Stella. Still we should call her a normal small-town child, certainly until her last year in grammar-school. She had some difficulty with her studies that spring because of her eyes. Her lenses, fitted in Atlanta, seemed to make them worse. It was only after she went to a noted specialist in Charleston that she was relieved. It is significant that later these expensively obtained glasses were discarded as "too much trouble."

The summer Stella was thirteen, Grandmother Beckman came to spend her last days in her son's home. The granddaughter had been named for her, and Grandmother was frail and old and needed attention. Grandmother also had some means. For over a year the young girl gave much of her time to the old lady, and for over a year she was able to lead the Beckman table-talk with her wealth of details about Grandma's sickness. Stella's care of her charge was excellent, entirely lacking in any selfish element. Death hesitated, when he finally called, and for nearly a week the dying woman lay unconscious. These "days of strain" and the death and funeral were, always after, mentioned by Stella and her people as her "first shock." For a time she was so nervous and restless and her sleep so disturbed that the doctor gave her hypnotics and advised her being sent away. She went to Atlanta for two months, boarding in the home of a Methodist minister, who some years before had been stationed in Rome. It was Stella's first experience in a religious home. She had never been accustomed to hearing the "blessing" said, and food referred to as "God-given" seemed, at first, quite too sacred to swallow. And the effect of morning worship--the seriously read Bible chapter, the earnest prayer, with the entire family kneeling--affected her profoundly, and gave to this godly home a sanctity which, at susceptible not-yet-fifteen, awakened emotions so powerful that for days she walked as one in a dream, one attracted by some wonderful vision which was drawing her, unresisting, into its very self. Each day was a step closer, and at prayer-meeting the Wednesday night before she returned home, she announced her conversion, with an intensity of earnestness which could but impress every hearer.

Stella Beckman went back to Rome filled with a zeal for the new religious life which commanded the respect of even her religiously careless father. Nor was it a flash in the pan. She joined the church. She made her sister join the church, and to the church she gave four years of remarkable devotion. Church interests were first, and one Sunday the pastor publicly announced that for the twelve months past Stella Beckman had not missed a single service in any branch of the church's activities. She taught a Sunday-school class. She sang in the choir. She was president of the Epworth League, and not only attended, but always "testified" at mid-week prayer-meeting. Her church interests took all her time. The foreign-missionary cause later laid a gripping hold upon her, and arrangements were made, four years after she went into the church, for her to go to a Missionary Training- School.

Somehow things went wrong here. She had expected an almost sanctified atmosphere. She was accustomed to being regarded as essentially devout, but there was a sense of order in the school which she felt was mechanical, class-room work seemed to be counted as important as religious services, and her fervidly expressed religious experiences appeared to reflect chill rather than the accustomed warmth of the home prayer-meetings. Moreover, real lessons were assigned which no amount of religious feeling or no intensity of personal praying made easy. She hadn't studied for years; in fact, she had never learned to do intellectual work studiously. And even these good religious teachers did not hesitate to demand accurate recitations. She had been accustomed for years to have preference shown, and here she was treated only as one of many, and, humiliatingly, as one who was failing to maintain the standards of the many. She fell behind in the two most important studies, nor was her classwork in general good. Whether she would have later proven capable of getting down to rock bottom and meeting the demands of reason on a rational basis, we cannot say, for the family hobby abruptly terminated her missionary career. "Mother dangerously sick with inflammatory rheumatism. Come at once," the telegram said--and she hastily returned home to be met with, what her history records as, "my second shock." Her mother WAS sick, and truly and genuinely suffering. The house was in disorder. Weeks followed in which Stella's best strength was needed. Her mother slowly mended, but never regained her old activity. The doctor said a heart-valve was damaged, and the family thereafter were never quite certain when the sudden end would come--an uncertainty which was proven legitimate ten years later, when she died, almost suddenly. Stella had met shock number two very well. The home-love and welcome and the warmth of feeling she experienced in the home-church were a never-admitted relief from the rigid exactions of the training- school life, and did much to neutralize, for the time, her anxiety about her mother and the "strain of her care." It was a family which ever advertised home-devotion, and so this call of home illness completely obscured all other plans for three years. But home responsibilities quite wrecked her church-going record. In fact, it was unkindly whispered that Stella was "backsliding." And these same whispers found audible expression the summer she was twenty-two, when attractive Lee Burnham, the judge's son, spent his summer vacation at home, and "took her buggy-riding every Sunday evening for over two months."

Lee was only twenty-one, but his was a very romantic twenty-one, and he filled Stella's ears with so many sweet nothings that she no longer heeded the call of duty. And why shouldn't she be in love and have a lover? Had she not already given the best years of her youth to others? Had she not waited without a thought of rebellion for the coming of the right one? And Love, and Love's mysterious touch, wrought fantastic changes in Stella Beckman's affairs. She and Lee read poetry. She had never known how beautiful poetry was nor how much of it there was to read. He knew the good novels and sent her all that he himself read, and these were plenty! Then, when he was away, he wrote and she wrote, and now and then he wrote some verses to her. There was no real engagement. They never spoke much of the future; the present was too full. Home duties and church interests flagged badly during these two years, and the summer she was twenty-four, it became town talk that this young couple would marry. The Beckmans were very willing. But one day the judge called Lee into his office and wanted to know what these "doings" all meant, asking him if he was "going to marry his mother," and making some rather uncomplimentary Beckman- Burnham comparisons. Lee rather sheepishly told his father there was nothing to worry about. He had much respect, possibly awe, for the old gentleman. The next week Lee left for his final year in law-school. His letters to Stella continued, though he plead his studies as an excuse for their diminished frequency. He did not come home that spring, at Easter. "Work," he wrote Stella. Nor was he ever square to this poor girl, for he never mentioned his relations with Miss Pearl May Rogers. And "shock number three" came, as unhappy Stella read the announcement of his marriage, addressed in the hand of his June city- bride. A lastingly damaging shock it proved to be.

Stella was put to bed; for days she lay in deep apathy. Feeding became a problem of nurses and doctors. She cared for nothing--nothing "agreed" with her, and she lost weight rapidly. Chills and flushes, sweatings and shakings came in regular disorder, and for hours she would be apparently speechless. Somebody--not the doctors--reported that Stella Beckman had typho-malaria. Abnormal sensitiveness to surroundings, to sounds, sights and smells, especially a dread of unpleasant news, were to complicate her living for years to come. For the remainder of her life she was to confound sensations normal to emotional reactions with sensations accompanying physical diseases; and sensations came and went in her now tense emotional nature like trooping clouds on a stormy day. Stella's illness was so prostrating that her weakened mother and busy sister could not care for her adequately, and an aunt came to help. Recovery was slow and imperfect; she remained a semi-invalid for two and a half years. Physical discomforts were so constant that a surgeon was finally consulted who did an exploratory operation and removed some unnecessary anatomy. This man's personality was strong, his desire to help, genuine, and he had considerable insight into the emotional illness of his patient. The influence of the operation, with the surgeon's encouragement and the atmosphere of confidence pervading the excellent, small surgical hospital, combined to make Stella very much better for the time. But within less than three years, her father died. She calls this "the fourth shock," and it resulted in another period of nervous illness. She cried much at the time. Work was impossible--as was all exercise --because of her rapid fatigue. One day she slipped on the front steps and, apparently, but bruised her knee. Her doctor nor the X-ray could discover more serious damage. Still, walking was practically discontinued, as she could not step without pain. At last, almost in desperation, her brother took her to a hospital noted for its success in reconstructing nervous invalids. At this time she weighed but one hundred and four, and the list of her symptoms seemed unending. A desire to be helped, however, was discerned and with rest-treatment she gained rapidly in weight, appetite returned, digestive disturbances disappeared, and massage, or a new idea, fully restored her walking powers. She became eager for the more important half of her treatment--the out-of-door work-cure. During these weeks she had certainly been given much physical and mental help. Expert and specialized counsel and nursing had been hers.

At the end of five months Stella returned to Georgia--restored--a health enthusiast. It now became her joy, in and out of season, whenever she could secure hearers, to relate the details of her illness and the miracle of her restoration. The methods of the special hospital that wrought such wonders for her were reiterated in detail, and for years she made herself thoroughly wearisome by her talk of diet and exercise, special bathing, out-of-door work and prescribed habits. She kept herself constantly conspicuous in her efforts to reform others to her new ways of living. For over four years, she sedulously adhered to the routine outlined by the hospital, with such devotion to, and augmentation of, details that she had little time for church and practically no time for household affairs. As had been her habit in past experiences her enthusiasm was causing her to overdo, and the business of keeping well seemed now her only object in life. This could not go on interminably. Something had to happen, and her mother's rather sudden death proved the shock which was to relieve her from the overenthusiastic slavery to an impracticable routine.

Stella Beckman at forty-five is sadly less fine and worthy than the Stella Beckman of eighteen. Religion, Love and Science have each entered her life deeply to enrich it, but all of these built upon the sands, the shifting sands of an emotional nature which had never laid the granite foundation of reason. Since the mother's death, the logic of her feelings has become more and more crippled by false valuations. She lives at home keeping house for the boys, recounting each mealtime the endless list of her feelings; bringing herself, her sickness, her hospital experiences wearisomely into the conversation with each caller. The emotional stability and the will to persevere even at considerable cost, which marked youth, are gone. At forty-five her life is objectlessly spasmodic, the old family-habit of talking of self and the family-fetish of discussing sickness have honeycombed her character and made her hopelessly tiresome. And her feeling-life is as restless as a troubled sea.

CHAPTER XIII

WILLING ILLNESS

Mr. Harrison Orr lived till he was twenty-five in Indianapolis, the town of his birth, excepting the years spent in Chicago pursuing his literary and law courses. He inherited a small fortune and, after two years spent in "seeing the world," located in Memphis, Tennessee. Here, as an attorney and later as an investor, he was professionally, financially and socially successful. His father had been liberal in the use of wines and cordials, and young Orr himself always remained a "good fellow," just the kind of a man to attract a vivacious, socially proud daughter of the South. He was thirty-five when he married-- accounted an age of discretion. His experience with womankind was so ample that he should have made no mistake in his final, irrevocable choice, and, be it said to his honor, no one, not even the wife herself, ever knew by word or act of his, to the contrary. He and his Mississippi bride spent thirty years in apparent domestic tranquillity, until he died at sixty-five from a heart which refused longer to have its claims for purposeful living eternally answered by gin rickeys and nips of "straight Scotch."

Mrs. Harrison Orr is unconsciously the unhappy "villain" of our tale. Her girlhood home was on a large sugar-plantation where she, as an only child, was reared to dominate her surroundings, while her parents made particular effort that she might shine socially. Parts of many years she lived in Washington in the home of a political relative, and attended a select girls' school. After her debut she spent the social winters at the Capitol where social niceties were developed with much attention to detail, and at home and while in Washington she was gratifyingly popular. "A brilliant conversationalist," she had heard herself called when fifteen, and the art of conversation, hitherto far from neglected, became by choice and practice her forte. Brilliancy in speech ever remained her only seriously attempted accomplishment. Clever of speech, from childhood, she had early learned to utilize this ability to attain any desired end. And talk she could, and talk she did, and as she grew older, by sheer talking she domineered every situation. It was her opinion when she married that at any time, with any listener, she could talk cleverly on any subject. As the years passed, during which she added little to her asset of knowledge, this art of fine speech gradually, but relentlessly, degenerated, and step by step she slipped down the paths of delicacy and fineness, through the selfishness of her insistent talkativeness.

Harrison Orr never intimated that his evenings at home were hours of boredom, but in later years spent much time in the comparative quiet of his club. Few intellects can be so amply stored as to continue brilliant through decades of much speaking, and the sparkle of Mrs. Orr's conversation was gradually shrouded in the weariness of what a blunt neighbor termed her "inveterate gabble." As it must be, this woman of exceptional opportunities early lost true sensitiveness, and, both as guest and hostess, ignored the offense of inconsiderate and self- seeking interruptions. She broke into the speech of others with crude abandon. The itch to lead and preempt the conversation became uncontrollable. Finer natures thrown with her could but tolerate her "naive" discourtesy, while dependents had to dumbly endure. Mrs. Orr but stands as a type illustrating far too many mortally wearisome, social pretenders, prominent only through the tireless tiresomeness of their much speaking.

The wreckage which may follow a single unthought crudity, in a home otherwise exceptional, is signally illustrated in the life of Mrs. Orr's only child, Hortense, born two years after their marriage. From the first she was sensitive and high-strung, nervously damaged probably in her early years by her mother's restless, unwise overcare. When Hortense was five she was sharply ill for several weeks with scarlatina. During these days she was isolated with Mrs. Place, her nurse, in a wing of the home. As fortune would have it, Mrs. Place was the daughter of a rural English clergyman. After the death of her husband, who left her limited in means, she came to America, where she trained. Her wholesome influence over Hortense, her general demeanor in the home, and her many excellent qualifications as nurse and woman attracted Mr. Orr's discerning attention, and he induced her to remain as governess to his daughter. Mrs. Place proved a most excellent addition to the Orr household. Always deferential, she was never servile; always reserved, she ever faced duties large and small, promptly, quietly and efficiently. Never, through her nearly ten years as daily companion of Hortense, did her speech or conduct betoken aught but refinement. More and more Hortense retreated to her wholesome companionship in face of the assaults of her mother's trying volubility. In many ways this most unusual nurse protected her charge from the greater damage of poor mothering than actually occurred. The differences between these two women were reflected in the sensitive child's life. Unconsciously at first, later in certain details, ultimately without reserve, she approved the standards of the one and repudiated those of the other. In contrast to her mother she grew into an abnormal reserve.

Hortense never attended the public schools but was regularly taught by Mrs. Place until she was fifteen, when she went East and entered her mother's old school, in Washington. The years of her careful tutoring had failed to accustom her to competition of any kind, and this first year of school work was taxing and but indifferently successful. During the spring term she had measles which left her with a hacking cough, and she did not regain her lost weight. The school-doctor sent her home, "for the southern climate," where she remained for a year, rather frail and the object of much detailed, maternal solicitude. It was probably this same solicitude which finally became so wearying that she returned to school for relief. Hortense was now a year behind, but resented the rather superior airs of some of her old classmates so effectively that she got down to business, made up her back work, and graduated reasonably well up in her entrance class. Of light build, and always frail in appearance, she did commendable work in school athletics. She took private instruction in hockey, for she was determined "to make the team," and her success in accomplishing this is significant of her ability to do, when she willed. At one of the later inter-scholastic games she met a handsome, manly, George Washington University student. She was nineteen, he twenty-three, and on his commencement day he honored her by offering his hand. Her southern love was aglow. Her lover was practically making his own way, but his prospects were excellent, his character superior, and they both cared very much.

Unhappily, Mrs. Place had returned to England, or Hortense would have confided in her and some futures might have been different. But the warmth of the new love seemed at the time to dissipate the chilliness toward her mother, which, unexpressed to herself, had through the years been increasing in the daughter's heart. So she wrote a long letter full of the beautiful story of the growing happiness, with pages of fervid descriptions of a certain fine young fellow, and importuned her mother to come East at once and to bring her blessing. No such filial warmth had Mrs. Orr ever before known. No such opportunity for a beneficent expression of the high privilege of motherhood had ever been entrusted to her. She responded without hesitation. She did not even wait to read their daughter's letter to her husband. When she reached Washington she summoned the young suitor to her hotel, and succeeded in one masterful quarter of an hour in arousing his violent dislike and lasting contempt. Through diplomacy she got Hortense on the Memphis-bound train. She was determined that her "darling child" should never marry beneath her station, and she talked and talked, drowning her daughter's protests, appeals and objections, in her merciless flow of words. Night after night she would stay with her till after twelve, leaving the poor girl tense, distracted and sleepless. And the habit of sleeplessness developed and with it a painfully abnormal sensitiveness to noises. The cruelly disappointed girl rapidly went to pieces. She craved a woman's sympathy, she longed for a mother's comprehending love, but she soon came to dread even her mother's presence, and formed the habit of burying her ears in the pillows to shut out the sound of that voice which could have meant the sweetest music of all, yet which to her distraught nerves had become an irritating, repelling, hated noise. Then special nurses came; the hot months were spent in the Rockies; several sea-trips were made; twice patient and nurse went East to forget it all in weeks of concerts and theaters in New York. But her inability to sleep was but temporarily relieved, while her antagonism to noises increased. She was then in Philadelphia for six months under the care of a noted neurologist, where she slowly gained considerably, physically, and was sufficiently well to spend a short, social "coming out season" with her parents. Yet the "at homes" and tea-parties and functions in which her mother reveled, never more than superficially interested her.

Rather strangely, father and daughter had not been as close as their similar natures and needs would suggest. While Mrs. Orr may not have been jealous, she preempted her husband's home hours mercilessly; but in her father's death Hortense came to know that one of the few props of her stability had been removed. Moreover, her mother's incessant reiteration of her loneliness and sorrow, and the endless discussion of the details of her depressing widow's weeds, and of her taxing, exhausting widow's responsibilities, brought on a return of the old symptoms, with the antipathy to noises even intensified. We may think of Hortense Orr as inherently weak. This is not so. Save as influenced in her girlhood by Mrs. Place, and while stimulated during her last three years at school by personal ambition, she had known no duties nor responsibilities. There had never been any necessity for specific effort or sacrifice. After her great disappointment she had surrendered to depression of spirit, and she reacted in the same way after her father's death. And this surrender was early followed by weakness of her disused body. She also surrendered to the weakness of self-pity, that craven mocker of self-respect. She was not a will-less girl, but life had brought her small chance to develop that will which masters, while wilfulness, that will which demands selfishly for self, grew out of the soil so largely of her mother's preparing. This wilfulness, first asserted in small things, grew and grew.

The family doctor saw more than tongue and liver and thin blood and bodily weakness. He realized the helplessness of Hortense in finding her stronger self in the home atmosphere, and advised a year in Europe--to get away from her sorrow, he said, to get away from her mother's wearying discussion of details, he knew. For nearly a year she was treated in Germany at different cures without benefit. It was always the "noise" that kept her from sleeping. It was the "noise" which she had learned to hate and to revile. To get away from noise became her fixed determination. And to this end a small mountain- cottage was secured, secluded from the haunts and industries of man, in the remoteness of the Tyrolean Alps. Here with her nurse and a servant she remained three years. For the first months she seemed happier, and took some interest in the inspiring views and rich flora of her surroundings. But the night did not bring the silence she willed. She sensed the heavy breathing of her nurse, the movements of the servant as she turned in her bed, and sometimes even snored, she knew it! She would spend hours of strained, sleepless attention, alert to detect another instance of the heartless repetition of this incriminating sound. She must be alone. She feared nothing so much as the hated sounds of human activity. So a one-room shack was built a hundred yards away from her companions, in the deeper solitude of the forest. Here she slept alone, month after month. But the winters, even in the Tyrolean foot-hills, are severe at times, and the deadly monotony of this useless life, and the improvement which she "knew" would come with the perfection of her sleeping arrangements, combined to decide her to return home, though still an enemy to the unbearable sounds of the night. Twenty-eight years she had lived with no true interest in life; neither home, attractions in New York or in Europe, nor treatment offered by competent and kind specialists had influenced her one thought away from her willingness to be ill. The nurse, who had buried herself so long with this poor girl in Europe, was quite appalled at Mrs. Orr's inconsideration of her daughter's "sensitive, nervous state." Nurse and mother soon had words; nurse and daughter left promptly for the East, where two hours from New

York they spent another year in semi-isolation together.

A New York broker owned the place adjoining the invalid's cottage. Walter Douglas, then but twenty-six, was his private secretary. Walter and Hortense met in the quiet, woodland paths. It is difficult to know just what the mutual attractions were. She had received many advantages which had not been his, still life was certainly a lonely thing for her. He was her first real interest since she had left Washington, and love reawakened and blew into life the embers she thought were gray-cold. It was never to be the flaming love-fire of ten years before, but it was bright enough to decide her to marry, which she did without writing any letter of confidence to her unsuspecting mother.

Mr. Orr had left the property in his wife's control, and she had been unquestionably most generous in supplying her daughter with funds. When she received the brief note telling of the little wedding and inviting her to meet them in Washington, on their simple wedding-trip, she found herself for the first time in her life--speechless! There were no words to express this "outrage." The disability was short- lived, but her letter to the bridal couple was shorter. They had taken things into their own hands; they had ignored her who had every right to be at least advised, and they could take care of themselves. Hardly had this letter been mailed when she consulted her attorney as to ways and means to annul this "crazy marriage."

The young couple had more pride than dollars, and bravely started house-keeping in a small flat. Few had been more inadequately trained for household duties than this self-pampered woman who pluckily at first, then grimly, went to the limit of her poorly developed strength in an effort to make homelike their few, plain rooms, and to prepare their unattractive meals. Still it all might have worked out had the noises of the street not attained an ascendancy. In less than four months the youthful husband, through a sense of duty, wrote the mother details of his bride's "precarious condition." Mrs. Orr promptly sent money, and the mother in her soon brought her to them in person. Within a few days she recognized the helpless husband's honesty and patience, and took them both to Memphis, providing a furnished flat and a good servant. The incompetent wife's short experience in household responsibilities, for which she was so utterly unprepared, made sickness a most welcome haven of refuge, and for months she did nothing but war with the noises of the quiet suburb. Then their baby came, but with it slight evidence of young mother love. She seemed almost indifferent to her little one. At rare times, only, would she respond to her first-born and to her husband. The doctor said there was no reason why she did not regain strength, that she could if she would, that it was not a question of physical frailty but it was decidedly a case of willing to have the easiest way. "Something has to be done," he said at last, and he strongly advised that she be sent to a hospital where she would be the object of benevolent despotism. She constantly complained of her oversensitive hearing, and had certainly developed all the arts of the invalid. She made no objection to the proposed plan. She did not know what was in store for her, outside of the mentioned "rest-cure." Full authority was given the institution officials to use any possible helpful means to stimulate her recovery. In all this the family physician counseled wisely and with discernment. At the hospital Hortense Douglas was told that she was to remain until she was well, that it was not a question of duration of treatment, but of her condition, which would determine the date of her return to her home, husband, and little one. The relationship between her years of illness and her unhappy disappointment, between her antagonism to night sounds and her intolerant impatience with her mother, was carefully explained. The ideal of making friends with these same noises which were but the voices of human progress, happiness, industry and personal rights, was held before her. Following the first clash of her will with the hospital authorities, she claimed that she was losing her mind, and was told that she would be carefully watched and would be treated at once as irresponsible when she proved to be so. Step by step she was forced to health, she was compelled to live rationally. Scientific feeding produced rapid improvement in her nutrition, she gained strength by the use of foods which she had never liked, had never taken and could "not take." In every way she improved in spite of herself. She often said she could not stand the treatment. But cooperation relentlessly proved more pleasant than rebellion. At the end of five months she was sleeping night after night the deep sleep honestly earned by thorough physical weariness, a sleep which nervous tire and worrying apprehension can never know. She could get no satisfaction as to when she would be allowed to return home.

She had no money in her possession, but she slipped away one morning, pawned her watch for railway-fare, and arrived home announcing that she was well.

Wealth, medical experts, years in Europe, society, the pleasures of seasons in New York, a husband's love, motherhood had failed to find health for this wilful woman. Not until her illness was made more uncomfortable than the legitimate duties of health, not until she recognized it was normal living at home or life in that "awful hospital," did she will to be well--and well she was.

CHAPTER XIV

UNTANGLING THE SNARL

You have probably passed the mansion. It stands, prominent, on the avenue leading from Buffalo to Niagara Falls. Three generations have added to its beauty and appointments. A generation ago it stood, imposing, and if fault could be found, it was its self-consciousness of architectural excellence. Every continent had contributed to its furnishings, and some of its servants, too, were trained importations. In the middle eighties, this noble pile was the home of an invalid, a twelve-year-old boy, a housekeeping aunt, and nurses, valets, maids, butlers, cooks, and coachmen. The invalid master of the house was forty-eight. As he leaned on the mantel looking out across the lawn, you felt the presence of a massive, powerful physique, but as he slowly turned to greet you, you fairly caught your breath from the intensity of the shock. The cheeks were hollow; the lips were ever parted to make more easy the simple act of breathing, the pallor of the face was more than that of mere weakness--there was a yellowish hue of both skin and eye-whites. The shrunken claw-like hands that offered greeting, the shrunken thighs, the increased girth of body which had so deceived your first glance, all bespoke mortal illness to even the untrained eye--advanced cirrhosis of the liver, to the professional scrutiny. And he was to be the fourth, in a line of financially successful Kents, to die untimely from mere eating and drinking. You would not have stayed long with this sick man. Only a large love or a large salary could have made the atmosphere of his presence endurable, for he was the essence of impatience, the quintessence of wilfulness. The sumptuousness of his surroundings, the punctilious devotion of his servants, the deferential respect shown him in high financial circles, books, people, memories, all failed ever to soften that drawn, hard face, for he was a miserably wretched, unhappy sufferer. Now and then his eyes would light up when Francis, his son and heir, was brought in. But Francis had a governess and an aunt who were respectively paid and commanded to keep him entertained and contented, and to see that he did not long disturb the invalid. That last year was one of most disorderly invalidism--not disorder of a boisterous, riotous kind, but an unmitigated rebellion to doctors' orders and advice, to the suggestions of friends, to the urgings and pleadings of nurses and "Aunt Emma." There were no voluble explosions; the impatience was not of the noisy kind--he had too much character for that, but the stream of thought was turgid and sulphurous. Jan, the valet, never argued, urged, suggested--by no little foreign shrug of his shoulders did he even hint that the master's way was not entirely right--and politic, faithful Jan stood next to Francis in his good graces; in fact, he was more acceptable as a companion. The only reason the sick man gave for his indifference to professional advice was that he was the third generation to go this way--and this way he went. A giant he was in the forest of men, felled in his prime.

Francis did not know his mother. She had been beautiful, a gentle, lovable daughter of generations of social refinement. Her father and grandfather had lived "pretty high." In truth, had the doctors dared, "alcoholic," as an adjective, would have appeared in both their death certificates; and the worm must have been in the bud, for she died suddenly at twenty-five, following a short, apparently inadequate illness. Thus, three-year-old Francis was left to a busy father's care, a maiden aunt's theoretical incompetence, and to the ministrations of a series of governesses who remained so long as they pleased their youthful lord. The undisciplined father's idea of good times, for both himself and his son, was based upon having what you want right now, and why not?--with unlimited gold, with its seemingly unlimited buying power. Dear Auntie, poor thing! knew no force higher than "Now, Francis, I wouldn't," or "Please don't," or on very extreme occasions, "I shall certainly tell your father"--as utterly ineffective in introducing one slightest gleam of the desirability and potency of unselfishness into this boy's mind, as was the gracious servility of the servants.

Francis was large for his age, unusually active and remarkably direct mentally, therefore little adjustment was needed as he entered that usually leveling community--boy-school-life. He was generous and good- hearted to a lovable degree and with such qualities and advantages he early became, and remained, leader in his crowd. After his father died, the boy, not unnaturally, placed him--the only one whose will he had ever had to respect--high in his reverence. The father had been a powerful young man, a boxer to be feared, oar one in the Varsity Crew; a man who, through the force and brilliancy of his business life, had won more than state-wide prominence, and had left many influential friends who spoke of him in highest respect. It was to be expected that the father's strong character would have deeply influenced his only son, and like father like son, only more so, he grew. But the "more so" is our tale.

"Rare, juicy tenderloin steaks go to muscle. You don't need much else, and we didn't get much else at the training-table," the father used to say, and they unquestionably formed the bulk of the boy's naturally fine physique, for he developed in spite of much physical misuse into a two-hundred-pound six-footer. Francis began smoking at twelve. On his tenth birthday a small wine glass had been filled for him and thereafter he always had wine at dinner, and he liked it--not only the effects but the taste. The desire was in his blood--Before he was eighteen he was brought home intoxicated and unconscious. No law had ever entered into his training which suggested any form of self-control. The principles of self-mastery were unthought; they had been untaught. "Eat, drink and be merry" might express the sum of his ideals. And so, physically or mentally, no thought of restraint entered his youthful philosophy. There was nothing vicious, no strain of meanness, much generosity; naturally kindly and practically devoid of any spirit of contention, and peculiarly free from any touch of the disagreeable, he was blessed with a spirit of good fellowship. He never questioned the rights of his friends to do as they pleased, and they quite wisely avoided questioning his right to do likewise; so, desire was untrammeled and grew apace. It was in Francis Kent's failure to bridle this power that the threads were first snarled.

The boy's fine body was trained in a haphazard way. Had his father lived, it might have been different. Mentally, he was naturally industrious and next to the joys of the flesh came his studies. It was as toastmaster at his "prep-school" commencement-banquet that he first drank to intoxication. The next fall he entered Yale, and there is no question but those days this revered university had a "fast set" that was emphatically rapid. But Francis Kent could go the paces; in fact, none of the football huskies could put in a night out and bring as snappy an exterior and as clear a wit to first class next morning as young Kent. His heredity, his beefsteaks, the gods, or something, certainly made it possible for him to be a "bang-up rounder" and at the same time an acceptable student through four college years.

He was almost gifted in a capacity for the romance literatures, and, anomalous though it may seem, he majored and excelled in philosophy. He was truly a popular fellow when he took his degree at twenty-two. High living had given him high color; his eye was active and his face, though somewhat heavy, was mobile with the sympathy of intelligence; his physique was good; he dressed with a negligee art which was picturesque. Big of heart, he had a wealth of scholarly ideas, and not a few ideals; many thought he faced life a certain winner.

Practically every door was open to him, and he chose--Europe. Those were two hectic years. Every gait was traveled; for weeks he would go at top-speed, go until nerve and blood could brook no more. No conception of the duty of self-restraint ever reached him till, at last, the nervous system, often slow to anger, began to express its objection to the abuse it was suffering. He was not rebounding as in the past from his excesses. For a day or so following a prolonged drinking bout he would be apprehensive and depressed, unable to find an interest to take him away from the indefinite dread which haunted him. Not till he could again stand a few, stiff glasses of brandy could he find his nerve. A friend found him thus "shot up" one day and suggested that he was "going the pace that kills," and hinted that another path might be trod with wisdom. "What's the use?" Kent flung back, "I'm fated to go with an alcoholic liver; it's in the family strong--both sides. I saw my father go out with it. I know Mendel's theory by heart, two black pigeons never parent a white one." And on he went. His creed now might well have been: "For to-morrow I die."

It may have been the impulse of an unrecognized fear--he said it was philosophic interest--which had attracted him to study the various theories of heredity. He had been particularly impressed by Mendel's "Principles of Inheritance," and its graphic elucidation of the mathematical recurrence of the dominant characteristics had grasped him as a fetish. With such forebears as his, there was no hope. The die had been cast before he was born. Why struggle against the laws of determinism? He was what he was because forces beyond his control had made him so. Scientific certainty now seemed to add its weight of evidence to his accepted fatalism, when, at twenty-eight, instead of the accustomed days of depression, a period of particularly heavy drinking was followed by a serious attack of delirium tremens. For several days he was cared for as one dangerously insane. After reason had been restored, the doctor, in his earnest desire to help, warned him that he must live differently and, knowing the father's ending, thought to frighten him into a change of habits by stating that his drinking would kill him in a few years if he kept it up. "You are already in the first stages of cirrhosis," he told him. As it turned out, no warning could have been less wise; it simply assured Kent the certainty of the fate which pursued, and soon he was at it again. Before thirty he had suffered two attacks of alcoholic delirium, had been a periodic drinker for fifteen years, a regular drinker for five years, often averaging for weeks two quarts of whiskey a day, and always smoking from forty to fifty cigarettes. Life had become more and more unlivable when he was not narcotized by alcohol or nicotine, and he was fast becoming a pitiful slave to his intoxicated and damaged nervous system.

He was living at home now, nominally secretary of a strong corporation-- practically eating, smoking, drinking, theater-going, lounging at the Varsity Club, and playing with his speedy motorboat. He enjoyed music and, when in condition, occasionally attended concerts. Barely he went to the Episcopal service, then only when special music was given. The faithful will discern the hand of Providence in his first seeing Martha Fullington in one of these rare hours at church. She was truly a fine, wholesome woman. The daughter of a small town Congregational minister of the best New England stock, she had always been healthy in body and mind. She possessed an unusual contralto voice, and came to Buffalo at twenty-two for special training. Helpful letters of introduction, with her pleasing self and good voice, rapidly secured her friends and a position in a fashionable church-choir. Here Kent heard her in a short but effectively rendered solo. Unsusceptible as he had been in the past, the sacredness of her religiously inspired face appealed to him strangely. Within a fortnight a new and profound element was to complicate his life, for he met Miss Fullington and took her out to dinner at the home of a classmate, whose mother was befriending the young singer. The spell of her charm wakened the power of his desire. Whether it was from the stimulation of her inherent difference to other women he had known, or whether deep within, and as yet untouched, there was a fineness which instinctively recognized and responded to fineness, we may not say with certainty. He was remote from her every standard, she thought, and her seeming indifference was a conscious self-defense. But she inspired him with a sincerity of purpose he had not known before. He was frank; he was potently insistent and "hopeless," he told her, "unless you save me." Thus unwittingly he appealed to the mother sympathy, the strongest a good woman can feel.

They were engaged and the wedding was all that any bride could have desired. Then ten weeks abroad, beautiful, revealing weeks, for Francis Kent, sober and in love, was much of a man. Still it was only ten weeks before the formal social function, with its inevitable array of wines, turned this kindly, genial lover, in an hour, into a coarse, inconsiderate drunkard. Confined for a week in their state-room on the steamer home with her husband, now a beast in drink, this poor, pure, uninitiated wife realized purgatory. Dark days were those next three years for them both. When sober, he was self-abased by the knowledge of the suffering of this woman he so truly loved, or was restlessly striving against desires which only alcohol could sate; while she was alternately fearing the debauch or fighting to keep her respect and love intact through the debauchery. For him, the battle waged on between love and desire, his love for her--his one inspiration, while desire was constantly reenforced by the taunts of his godless fatalism and the dead weight of his hopelessness.

Then came the day which is hallowed in the lives of even the ignorant and coarse, the day in which the young wife gladly suffers through the lengthening hours and goes down to the verge of the Dark River, that in her nearness to death she may find that other life, the everlasting seal of her marriage. In all the beauty of eagerly desired motherhood, Martha Kent bore her baby-boy. The father was not there. She did not then know all. They shielded her. He had been taken the night before to a private asylum, entering his third attack of delirium tremens, and while his wife in pain and prayer made life more sacred, he, struggling and uncontrolled, beast-like, was making life more repulsive. The pain of her motherhood never approached the agony of her wifehood, when she knew, while the pride of fatherhood was utterly submerged in the poignancy of his self-abasement, when he realized.

Another physician had treated him during this attack. He, too, wished to help. He talked with the humiliated man most earnestly, insisting that he had never truly tried, that in the past he had depended on his weak will and the inspiration of his devotion. He had not had scientific help. He assured him that he did not have incurable hardening of the liver and expressed, as his earnest belief, that there were places where the help he needed could be given--that there was hope. Plans were made and Francis Kent gave his pledge, expressed in a voluntary commitment, to carry out a six months' system of treatment. "Not," as he assured the physician-in-charge, "that I can be saved from the effects of what has gone before. I know my heredity is too strong for that. But by every obligation of manhood I owe my wife and boy five years of decent living. If you can make that possible, I shall be satisfied." The professional help Kent received, physically, was deep-reaching. It accurately adjusted food to energy expended. Forty self-indulgent cigarettes were transformed into three manly cigars, and he was put to work with his hands--those patrician hands which had not made a brow to sweat, for serious purpose, in three generations. His physical response in six weeks completely altered his appearance. The snap of healthy living reappeared; the pessimism of his fatalism was displaced by much of quiet cheer. Life was again becoming a good thing. But the professional help he received mentally was what untangled the snarl. His advisor was fortunately able to go the whole way with him as he discussed his hereditary "inevitables"--the whole way and then, savingly, some steps beyond-- and for the first time Kent's understanding, now reaching for higher truths than would satisfy the fatalist, was wisely, personally conducted through a wholesome interpretation of the distinction between the heritage of germinal and of somatic attributes, that vital distinction: that it takes but two ancestors to determine the species of the offspring, but that the individual's personal heritage is the result of, and may be influenced by, a thousand forerunners; that dominant characteristics, compelling though they seem, may be neutralized by obscure, recessive characteristics. More than this, his new counselor was able to convince him that the real damage he had to overcome was not a foreordained physical fate, for that was in a peculiar way largely in his own hands, now that he was properly started, but was the mental tangle of his unholy fatalism which absolutely did not represent truth; that he and all rational, normal men have been given wills and are as free as gods to choose, within certain large limitations. Francis Kent's mind had been well trained. Selfish desire had made of him a fatalist. A more beautiful desire led him into a constructive optimism. He thought deeply for a week, perchance he prayed, for he knew that she was praying from the depths of her soul. He outlined for himself a new, thoroughly wholesome mode of life, and in half an hour's heart-to-heart conference convinced his doctor-friend that more had been accomplished in two months than could have been promised at the end of the six months planned. So the new Francis Kent was told to go back and make a new home for his wife and the new baby. Years have passed--blessed years in the old mansion. There is no hint of cirrhosis of the liver. There has never been a drop of anything alcoholic served in that house since his return. There are two healthy chaps of boys; there is a wonderfully happy woman; there is a fine, manly man, the respected and efficient president of an influential bank. Patient, wise hands carefully untangled the knotted snarl. The thread was unbroken.

CHAPTER XV

FROM FEAR TO FAITH

Thirty some years ago a baby girl came into a Virginia home. Her birth was a matter of family indifference; not specially needed, she was not particularly wanted. Her father, reared in a small town, having attained only moderate success as combination bookkeeper, cashier and clerk in a general store, could not enthuse over an arrival which would increase the burden of family expense. He was a man of good Virginia stock, not fired by large ambitions. An ubiquitous cud of fine-cut, flattening his cheek and saturating his veins, possibly explains his life of semicontent--for tobacco is a sedative. The mother was a washed-out, frail-looking reminder of youthful attractions, essentially of the nervous type. She was not without pride in her Cavalier stock and the dash of Cavalier blood it brought. The elder sister had none of her mother. Aspiring socially, she was reserved, pedantic, platitudinizing, thoroughly self-sufficient. She finished well up in her class in a small, woman's so-called "college" and lived with such prudence and exercised such foresight that, in spite of her Methodist rearing, she wedded the young, local, Episcopal rector, and, childless but still self-sufficient, "lived happy ever after."

Our little Virginia's home surroundings gave her all material necessities, many comforts and occasional luxuries, but it was a home of narrow interests. Its own immediate affairs, including big sister's successes; critically, the doings of the neighborhood, and unquestioningly, the happenings of the church circle, comprised the themes of home discourse. Markedly lacking in beauty was that home--no music, a few perfunctory pictures, a parlor furnished to suit the local dealer's taste and stock, a few sets of books--the successful contribution of unctuous book agents. All converse was lacking in ideals save the haphazard ones brought home by the children from school. There was no pretense of unselfishness, the conception was foreign to that home's atmosphere. The religious teaching was of formalism and fear. The services of the church were regularly attended, and from time to time the children's discipline was augmented by references to the certain wrath of God. Into this home came Virginia to be reared under most irregular training, dependent on a combination of her mother's feelings and her sister's conventions-- the father's influence was negative, his was a well-bred nicotine indifference. In the little girl's life, every home appeal was emotional. During the mother's more rare, comfortable days, she exacted few restrictions, but much more often fear methods marked her use of authority: fear of punishment, fear of the Invisible, and, from her sister, fear of "what folks will say" were the chief home influences molding this young life. Such appeals found in her sensitive nature a rich soil. No single consistent effort was ever made to substitute reason for emotional supremacy, as she developed. At times her feelings would run rampant--what was to keep them in order but disorganizing fear?--while too often her mother weakly rewarded Virginia's most stormy outbreaks by acceding to her erratic desires.

In one element did this home take pride. As true Virginians, the good things of the table were procured at any cost. Good eating was a pride--and rapid eating became the child's habit. Yet with all the sacrifices of time and effort, the richness of their table cost, and in spite of the fact that eating was ever in the forefront of family plans and efforts, no conception of the true art of dining was ever theirs.

At sixteen Virginia was attractive, with remarkably clear, olive skin, with hair, eyes and eyebrows a peculiarly soft chestnut. Fun-loving, thoughtless, vivacious, spasmodically aggressive, naturally athletic, capable of many fine intuitions, she finished the local high school with a good record, for she was mentally alert. Still most of her thinking was of the emotional type, and smiles were quick and tears were quick, and upon a feeling-basis rested her decisions. The tender- heartedness of a child never left her, and when trusted and encouraged she had always shown an excellent capacity for good work. She was essentially capable of intense friendships, under the sway of which no sacrifice was questioned, but her stormy nature made friendships precarious. Pervading her life was a large conscientiousness. Her fear-conscience was acute--never an unwholesome impulse but fear- conscience rebuked and tortured. Few bedtimes were peaceful to her, because at that quiet hour remorse, entirely disproportionate to the wrong, lashed her miserably. Her love-conscience, too, was richly developed, and for love's sake she would have become a martyr. Her duty-conscience was yet in its infancy and held weak council in her plans and rarely swayed her from desire.

After a year of normal-school training, she secured a primary grade in a near town school, and at nineteen, when she became an earner, there were two Virginias; the beautiful Virginia was a woman of appealing tenderness--body, heart and soul yearned for some adequate return of the richness of devotion which she felt herself capable of giving. Sentiment and capacity for love were unconsciously reaching out for satisfying expression, and the beauty of this tenderness shone forth to make appealing even her weaknesses. The other Virginia was a conglomerate of unhappy and harmful emotions--impatient in the face of small irregularities, frequently irritable to unpleasantness, and dominated by the false sensitiveness of unmerited pride. Under provocation, anger, quick-flaming, unreasonable and unreasoning, burned itself out in poorly restrained explosions--a quarter-hour of wrath, a half-hour of tears and a half-day of almost incapacitating headache. She was ambitious and had rebelled at her limitations, especially as she grew to realize the smallness and emptiness of the home-life. She resented her sister's superior attitude, her officious poise, her college-education authority. But the damning defect was the remorseless grip of fear on mind, body and spirit. Through ignorant training, she was afraid in the dark, even afraid of the dark; a morbid, cringing terror possessed her when she was alone in the night. Even the protecting safety of her own bed could not save her from the jangle of false alarms with which her imagination peopled the shadows. A second gripping dread--one all too common with harmfully taught, southern girls--was fear of negroes; a horrible, indefinite, haunting apprehension chilled her veins, not only when associated with them, but even more viciously when she was alone with her thoughts. And when added to these was her superstitious fear of the Lord, magnifying the evil of her ways, threatening, pervading, bringing no hint of Divine love, the preparation was ample for the forthcoming emotional chaos.

At twenty-eight she was a sick woman. Through devotion to the kindly principal of her school, a devotion not unmixed with sentiment, she had worked intensely; quick, interested, almost capable, she had worked and worried. School-discipline early loomed large as a rock threatening disaster, dragging into her consciousness a sinister fear of failure. Thirty little ones, from almost as many different homes, representing a motley variety of home-training, looked to her to mold them into an orderly, happy unit. Some of her little tots were as thorns in her flesh--she couldn't keep her arms from around others; while some afternoons the natural restlessness of them all set her head to throbbing wretchedly. Her own emotional life not having found order or calm, she from the first failed to develop either in her charges. Visitors became a dread. Her only solace was the short conferences she had with the principal after school. But to hear his step approaching during class-time frightened her cruelly. Her order was poor. He knew it. The visitors saw it. And the more she struggled to master the problem of school-discipline, the greater grew the menace of her own unorderly training. Within a few months she was translating her emotional exhaustion into terms of overwork. The penalty of unmerited food had produced an autotoxic anaemia, and she was pale and weepy, easily fatigued, sleeping poorly, with the boggy thyroid and overactive tendon reflexes so common in subacidosis. She had to give up her school. After six months' ineffectual resting at home, she entered a special hospital where, after some weeks of intensive treatment, her physical restoration was remarkable. The marriage of her sister and death of her mother closed the home, and she went to live with a widowed aunt, the aunt who had managed her household and her ministerial spouse to perfection. It was probably Paul's injunction alone which kept her from taking her complacent husband's place in the pulpit and delivering the sermons she had so literally inspired. Here was an atmosphere of sanctity, but still no hint of true, personal giving, no expression of willing sacrifice, and Virginia felt keenly this lack, for in the hospital she had had a vision. There she had seen suffering softened by gentleness, there empty lives were filled from generous hearts, and men and women inspired to make new and better starts. She had visioned the nobleness of giving--and the unanswered call of her mother-nature had responded. She was not fully well, she was not deeply living, she had never fulfilled the best of self, and she hungered for the hospital. Her aunt's conventional pride was echoed by the laws and the in-laws, and positive, later peremptory objections were urged against her entering nursing. Again the headaches returned, the physical expression of her emotional unhappiness, and finally, almost in recklessness, certainly in desperation, she cast her lot in the self-effacing demands of a student-nurse's life in a city hospital, far from family and friends.

How shall we tell of the next three years? Training, reeducation, evolution?-- some of all perhaps. They were years of much travail. Physical wholeness was won promptly through the wholesome habits of active, daily effort, routine, regularity and rational diet. There was suffering--months of suffering, under correction, for rebellion had long been a habit, and hospital discipline is military in character. But she had given her pledge, and fear-conscience and love-conscience were later augmented by duty-conscience, and she never seriously thought of deserting. Cheer expression is demanded in the nurse's relations with her patients, and irritability and impatience slowly faded through hourly touch with greater suffering; and the cheer habit grew into cheer feeling. The old storms of anger seemed incongruous in the imperturbable atmosphere of the hospital, moreover her dignity as a nurse could not be risked. Thus was she helped till the solidity of self-control made her safe. Her truly formidable battle was with fear --no one can know what she faced alone on night duty. Her dread of the dark was overcome painfully when through helpful counsel she gained an intelligent insight into her defect, and was inspired to apply for night duty in excess of her regular schedule. Later, at her own request, she performed alone the last duties for the dead, that she might put fear under her feet. Her dread of negroes gradually gave place to a better understanding of the race through the daily association of ministration on the ward, reenforced by personal confidence in her own strength and skill, growing out of a wholesome training in self-defense--a training her love for athletics and her growing understanding of her fear-weakness moved her to take on her off-duty time. She became competent; anxious to help, her fineness of intuition and her capacity for devotion with her vision of service made her in every way worthy. And finally her fear of the Lord was lost in a wholesome faith in His "Well-done!"

To-day, hers is a life of peace. Emotional instability and wretchedness have been displaced by habitual right feeling. Stabilizing her emotions has not impoverished, but enriched her nature. She has mastered the art of enjoying, for self-interests have expanded into love for service. To-day she is a capable, efficient, cheerful, wholesome, self-forgetting woman, filled with a faith in an able, worthy self--a God-given faith.

CHAPTER XVI

JUDICIOUS HARDENING

In the softened light of a richly furnished office two physicians were seated. It was the elder who spoke. Drawn and sad was his cleanly featured, tense face; his clear skin and slightly whitened, dark hair belied his nearly seventy years. He was the anxious, unhappy father of a sick, unhappy daughter, whom the nurse was preparing in an adjoining room for examination by Dr. Franklin, the younger physician. "I mean no discourtesy, Doctor, when I say that I don't believe any one understands my girl's case. Her brother and sister are healthy youngsters and have always been so. I may have taken a few drinks too many now and then, but few men of my age can stand more night-work or do more practice than I can, and I've about rounded my three-score and ten. Wanda was a perfect child. She is my oldest. Her mother did pet and spoil her, always humored her from the first, but she was a cheerful, bright little thing. She finished high school at fifteen and did a good year's study at Monticello. All her trouble seemed to start that spring when she was vaccinated. She had never had worse than the measles before. She didn't seem to know how to take sickness, though the Lord knows she's had plenty of chances to learn since her sore arm; and the school-doctor had to lance a small place, and this kept her away from Commencement where they had some part for her to do. She didn't get well in time to spend the month in Michigan with her room- mate, and she always said that if she could have had this trip she would never have been so bad. It was a mighty hard summer with me, too, that year, and probably I didn't notice her enough--anyway she's been a half-invalid these eighteen years. It's pain and tenderness in this nerve and then in that one, and she hasn't walked a whole mile in fifteen years because of her sciatica. I have sent her to Hot Springs, one summer she spent at Saratoga, and she has taken two courses of mud-baths. When she was twenty-six, she lived for four months in Dr. Moore's home. He and I were college-mates and he had been mighty good in treating rheumatic troubles. After awhile he decided it was her diet and she lived a whole year in B--- Sanitarium and she gained weight too, there, and hasn't eaten any meat to speak of nor drunk any coffee since. She often complains of her eyes but the specialists say they are all right, that that isn't the trouble. Two of the best surgeons in our part of the country have refused to operate on her even when I begged one of them to open her and see if he couldn't find out what was the matter. Three of her doctors have said it was her nerves, but I don't think any of them know. You know I don't mean to say anything that will reflect on your specialty, but you never did see a case of only nerves put a healthy young girl in bed and keep her there suffering so that I've had to give her aspirin a hundred times and even morphin by hypodermic to get her quiet, and off and on for five years she's had ten, and sometimes fifteen grains of veronal at midnight, nights when she couldn't get to sleep. If it's only nerves, then I've got a mighty heap to learn about nerves. I think in forty- five years practicing medicine a man ought to know enough about them to recognize them in his own family. But something's got to be done. Wanda's making a hospital of our home. We daren't slam a door, or her sister mustn't play the piano but her headaches start; and if Rosie boils turnips or even brings an onion into the house, it goes to Wanda's stomach and it takes a hypodermic to quiet her vomiting and a week to get over the trouble.

"That child of mine is just like a different creature from the fine little girl she was at twelve when my buggy turned over one night and broke my leg. Why, she nursed me better than her mother. She just couldn't do enough for me. That little thing would come down just as quiet as she could--sometimes every night--to see that that leg was all right and hadn't got twisted; while now she expects attention from everybody in the house and from some of the neighbors. She will even send for Rosie just when she is trying to get dinner started and keep her a half-hour telling just what she wants and how it's got to be fixed, then more often she'll just nibble at it just enough to spoil it for everybody else, after Rosie's spent an hour getting it ready for her. Tonics don't help her a bit. I've given her iron, arsenic and strychnin enough to cure a dozen weak women. She's always too weak to exercise, lies in bed two days out of three, reads and sometimes writes a letter or two. But before Christmas comes (you know she is mighty cunning with her fingers; she can sew and embroider and make all sorts of pretty, womanish things) she works so hard making presents that she's just clear done out for the next two months and won't leave her room for weeks. That's about all she does from one year's end to another, but complain of her sickness, and of late years criticize the rest of us and dictate to the whole household what they must do for themselves, and just out-and-out demand what she wants them to do for her. She really treats her stepmother like a dog, and often she is so disrespectful to me that I certainly would thrash her if she wasn't so sick. She was a fine child but her suffering has wrecked her disposition. She and the rest of us would be better off if she'd die. You see, Doctor, I haven't much faith left, but she's been bent so long a time on coming to you, and is willing to spend the little money her mother left her, to have her own way. Now, I am doctor enough to stand by you in what you decide if you say you can cure her, and if she gets well, I'll pay every cent of the bill, but if she don't, the Lord will just have to help us all, though I suppose I'll have to take care of her as long as she lives for she won't have a cent after she gets through with this."

Wanda Fairchild lay expectant on the examination table, pale, almost wan; her blue eyes, fair skin and even her attractive, curling, blonde hair seemed lusterless, save when her face lighted with momentary anticipation at some sound suggesting Dr. Franklin's coming. Much indeed of her feeling life had grown false through the blighting touch of her useless years of useless sickness. But genuine was her greeting. "Oh, Doctor, I am so glad to be here! You remember Mrs. Melton. You cured her and she has been well ever since, and for over two years I've been begging papa to bring me here, but he hasn't any hope. He's tried so hard and spent so much. Now you've got to get me well. They all say this is my last chance. I certainly can't endure these awful pains much longer. I know they're going to drive me crazy some day if something isn't done to stop them. Just look at my arms. That's where I bit them last night to keep from screaming out in the sleeper, for I wouldn't take any medicine. I wanted you to see me without any of that awful stuff to make me different than I truly am. You will surely cure me, won't you, Doctor, so I can go back home soon, as strong as Mrs. Melton is, and live like other girls, and have company and go to parties and dance and take auto-rides and have a good time before I get too old--or die? Oh, Doctor, you don't know what a horrible life I live! Every day is just torture. I suppose they do as well as they know at home, but not one of them, not even papa, has any conception of how I suffer or they would show more consideration. It is terrible enough to be sick when you are understood and when everybody is doing the right thing to help you. I know my trip has made me worse, for my spine is throbbing now like a raw nerve. It would be a relief if some one would put burning coals on my back. You know there's nothing worse than nerve-pains."

Dr. Franklin smiled quietly. How often he had heard poor sufferers hyperbolize their suffering! How keenly he could see the distinction between the real and the false in illness! How certainly he knew that such exaggerated rantings and wailings stood for illness of mind or soul, but not of body! The physical examination, nevertheless, was extremely thorough. Nothing can be guessed at in the intricate war with disease.

"Yes, I was happy as a child. Mother understood me; no one else ever has. She knew when I needed petting. I did well at school and really loved Myrtle Covington, my room-mate at the Sem. Just think, she married--married a poor preacher, but I know she is happy, for she is well and has a home of her own and three children. I don't see how they make ends meet on eighteen-hundred and no parsonage. You know we had a smallpox scare at the Sem. that spring and all had to be vaccinated. I scratched mine, or something, and for weeks nearly died of blood-poisoning. That is where my neuritis started. They had to lance my arm to save my life, and when you examined me I had to grit my teeth to keep from screaming out when you took hold of that cut place. You believe I am brave, don't you, Doctor? It hurts there yet, but I didn't want to disturb you in the examination. Do you think there is any chance for me, Doctor?"

At this point the physician nodded to the nurse, who left the room.

"And what else happened that summer?" he asked her kindly.

"Well, I was in bed over three months with my vaccination and my lanced arm, and I had a special nurse, and couldn't eat any solid food for days. They never would tell me how high my fever was; they were afraid of frightening me, but I wouldn't have cared. I used to wish I could die."

"Why, child, what could have happened to make a young, happy girl of sixteen wish to die? Was there something really serious that you haven't told?"

"Oh, Doctor, didn't papa tell you? No, I know he wouldn't. He probably don't know--he can't know what it cost me. Oh! must I tell you? Don't make me, Doctor! Oh, my poor head! Doctor, it will burst, please do something for it. Oh, my poor mamma! She loved me so much and she understood me, too." And tears came and sobs, and for a time neither spoke.

"Tell me of your mother," the doctor said.

Then the story, the unhappy story, whined out in that self-pitying voice which ever bespeaks the loss of pride--that characteristic of wholesome normal womanhood. Her parents had probably never been happy together. The spring she was in the Seminary, ill, her mother left home. There was a separation. That fall her father re-married, as did the mother later, who lived in her new home but a few months, dying that same winter. From the first, Wanda had hated her stepmother. "I despise her. I can never trust Father again. I can never trust any one and I loathe home, and I want to die. Please, Doctor, don't make me live. I have nothing to live for!"

Here was the woman's sickness--the handiwork of an indulgent mother who had never taught her daughter the sterling ideals of unselfish living. This mother had gone. A better trained woman had entered the home, but her every effort to develop character in the stepdaughter was resented. Illness, that favorite retreat of thousands, became this undeveloped woman's refuge. Year after year, sickness proved her defense for all assaults of importuning duty. Sickness, weakly accepted at first, later grew, and as an octopus, entwined its incapacitating tentacles about and slowly strangled a life into worthlessness.

"Your daughter will have to leave Alton for nine months. Six of these she will spend on a Western ranch; for three months she will work in the city slums. Miss Leighton will be her nurse and companion. Life was deliberately planned to develop wills. Miss Fairchild has lost the ability to will until, at thirty-four, she is absolutely lacking in the power to willingly will the effort which is essential to rational, healthy living. She is but a whimpering weakling, a coward who for years has run from misfortune. Your daughter must be turned from discomfort to duty, from pain to productive effort; her margin of resistance must be pushed beyond the suggestive power of the average headache, periodic discomfort, or desire for ease; she must learn to transform a thousand draining dislikes into a thousand constructive likes. Finally, we hope to teach her the hidden challenge which is brought us all by the inevitable. To-day she is more sensitive than a normal three-months-old baby. She must be judiciously hardened into womanhood."

We cannot say that the troubled father gathered hope from this, to him, unique exposition of the invalid's case, but sufficient confidence came to induce him to promise his loyal support to the "experiment" for the planned period of nine months. The patient rebelled. She had come "to be Dr.

Franklin's patient." She couldn't "stand the trip." She wouldn't "go a step."

Yes, it seemed cruel. Three days and nights they were on the sleeper; forty miles they drove over increasingly poor roads to the big ranch in the Montana foot-hills where everybody else seemed so well, so coarsely well, she thought. After the first week the aspirin and the veronal gave out and there was no "earthly chance" of getting more. Then when she refused to exercise, she got nothing to eat but a glass of warm milk with a slice of miserably coarse bread crumbed in, and the mountain air did make her hungry; and when she was ugly, she was left alone, absolutely alone in that dreary room, and even Lee, the Chinese cook, wouldn't look in the window when she begged him for something else to eat. How she did love Rosie those "weary days of abuse"! Miss Leighton was always polite, though she would not stay with her a minute when she got "fussy," but would be gone for an hour, visiting and laughing and carrying on with the men-folks in the big- room. She had seemed so kind before they left the East and she was kind now, at times when she had her own way, but she was being paid to nurse a sick girl, and she had no right to leave her alone for hours simply because she whined or refused to do her bidding on the instant. There was a young doctor there who could have helped her if he would, but he had no more heart than the rest, and when the nurse called him in to make an examination, he was as noncommittal as a sphinx and gave her no speck of satisfaction, only telling her to do what the nurse said. Bitter letters she sent home, but somehow they all were answered by Dr. Franklin, who wrote her little notes in reply which made her angry--then ashamed. Verbal outbreaks there were, and physical ones, too, a few times, which the nurse calmly and humiliatingly credited to her exercise-account and brought her more to eat, saying that scrapping was as healthful as work in making strength. But somehow, she couldn't hate Miss Leighton long, as behind all her "cruelty" Wanda realized that a thoughtful friendship was ever waiting. One day they took a drive; when four miles from the ranch-house something happened, and they were asked to get out. They stood looking off over the ever-climbing hills to those remote, granite castles of the far Rockies.

The team started, and as they turned, the driver waved his apparent regrets. They walked back--four miles. Wanda had not performed such a feat in nearly twenty years. She walked off her resentment, in truth she was a bit proud, and the nurse certainly did bring her a fine supper, the first square meal she had been given in Montana. This was the turning point.

Walking, riding, working, camping in the open, sleeping in smoke and drafts after long hikes, carrying her own blanket and pack--all became matters-of-course. From 96 to l30--nearly thirty-five fine pounds--she put on. She even learned bare-back riding, and wove a rug from wool she had sheared, cleaned, dyed and spun. Long since, she had realized that Miss Leighton had only been carrying out Dr. Franklin's orders. That fall they came East to Baltimore. She worked with Miss Leighton in the tenement districts. She saw Dr. Franklin weekly. He now explained the principles underlying her ruthless, physical restoration. She learned to recognize her years of deficient will- living. The doctor revealed to her, as well, her great debt to her home, explained to her now cleared mind the poverty of the love she had borne, and wakened her to the stepmother's true excellence of character. Her opened eyes saw the great tragedy of defective living as reflected in the lives of want and evil in those to whom she was daily ministering. Her life had been blest in comparison.

A message came that her stepmother was ill--could she come home and help? That day this girl put off childhood and took on womanhood. She returned to her family a new woman, a thoughtful, considerate woman, an almost silent woman--save when speech is golden; a woman who makes friends and who remembers them in a hundred beautiful ways, a working woman, a home-maker for a happier father, for an almost dependent stepmother; a woman who was scientifically compelled to exchange self-condoling weakness for strength, who, when strengthened against her will, chose and lives the worthy life of self-giving. We wish her well, this new woman, who is repaying to her home a debt of years.

CHAPTER XVII

THE SICK SOUL

"Oh, 'War,' you just must win! I know you will!" "Keep a stiff upper lip, Old Fellow, and give them the best you've got." "Watch your knees, Buddie dear, and don't let them shake. Just think of us before you start, and remember we're pulling for you."--"Yes! and praying for you," whispered Eva Martin, who was shaking his hand just as the conductor called, "All aboard." And as Warren Waring gracefully swung aboard the last Pullman, the entire senior class of Beloit High gave the school-yell, with three cheers and a tiger for "War Waring."

What occasion could be more thrilling to a susceptible, imaginative sixteen-year-old boy than this demonstration of the aristocratic peerage of youth? For a half-hour he had been the center of-- admiration and encouraging attention, the recipient of a rapid fire of well-wishing, of advice serious and humorous, and unquestionably the subject of not a few unspoken messages directed heavenward. The kindly eyes of the old Beloit station have looked out upon many a scene of enthusiastic greeting and hearty well-wishing, but rarely has it seen these good offices extended to one of more apparent merit than handsome Warren E. Waring. One of the National Temperance societies had been utilizing the promising declamatory powers of the high school students of the country, through a series of county, district and state competitions, to influence the public. The contest in Wisconsin had finally eliminated all but the select few who were to contest for the temperance-oratorical supremacy of the state, and for a gold medal, as large as a double eagle, which was to be awarded by judges from the University faculty. The good wishes and cheers, stimulating advice, and silent prayers at the Beloit station had all been inspired by enthusiasm and confidence and love for the unusually gifted comrade now leaving for the competition.

For nearly a generation Squire Waring had struggled manfully, kindly, quietly, on his little farm up Bock River, adding a little now and then to the farm-income by the all-too-infrequent fees derived from his office as justice-of-the-peace. If the Squire had been a better farmer and less interested in books, especially in his yellow-backed law-books, the eking might not have been so continuous; and if his good wife had not been snatched away, at untimely thirty-five, by one of those accidents which we call providential, leaving a forty-year- old father alone with a five-year-old boy, her good sense would undoubtedly have made times easier with the Squire. As it was, his sister came to be mother in this little home. Good, steadfast Aunt Fannie she was, a woman without a vision, who accepted what the day brought with religiously unquestioning thanks. But as the only son grew and his charms multiplied, as the evidence of his gifts became manifest, the impracticable father let slip all personal ambition. The dreams he had dreamed for himself were to be fulfilled in his son, who would increase, even as he decreased. So it was that on his boy's tenth birthday the father turned from his ambition of years, to represent his county in the state legislature, and after forty-five doubled the time and strength devoted to his less than a hundred acres. "There must be money for the boy's education," he told his sister Fannie, "even if you and I have to skimp for the rest of our days. He's got the making of a state senator." The father was mistaken only in that he so limited his boy's possibilities.

The Squire helped the little fellow in his studies, and he entered the second grade of the near-by Beloit High School the fall before he was fourteen. The train-schedule was so arranged that he could return home every night; though, whenever the Squire felt that the farm-work justified it, and there was no occasion for his honorable court, they would drive to town together. This was the Squire's one joy. And proud he was to share in acknowledging the greetings which came from all sides, even when they drove through the best part of town in the old buggy--to feel the universal popularity in which his boy was held. Then there was the added satisfaction of a minute's chat with some one of the teachers, for they all had praise, and never a word of censure. Enjoyment enough this dear man got from these irregular trips to town to lighten for weeks the, to him, unnatural farm-labor; while petty offenders appearing before his tribunal were dealt with almost gently after one of these adventures in happiness.

Many a wealth-sated father would have exchanged his flesh and blood and thrown in his bank-balance to boot, could he have looked forward to so worthy an heir as promised to bless Squire Waring. The boy seemed to have been born to meet life successfully, whatever its challenge. Strong almost to sturdiness, yet agile and accurate in movement, he had "covered all sorts of territory around 'short,' and could hit the ball on the nose when it counted," and to him went the unprecedented glory of a forty-yard run for a touch-down and goal in a High School vs. Varsity Freshmen game. His were muscles which seemed to have been molded by a sculptor's hand. His face was manly. His waving dark-brown hair, deep-blue eyes, strong nose and rarely turned chin, his unfailing good-nature, his unquestioned nerve, his mental keenness and clearness, his remarkable power of expression, whether in recitation, school-theatricals or at young people's meetings; his instinctive courtesy of greeting, his apparent openness and honesty of dealing, his fairness to antagonist on field and platform, above all, his devotion to his unquestionably rural father, had made Warren Waring a school hero, even a model, in a church college-town.

What other boy in Wisconsin was so well equipped to win the gold medal? Sixteen years and some months! A rather youthful lad to stand before a thousand strange faces, to be the object of professorial scrutiny, to listen to the exultant plaudits of local partisanship; not to be, not to seem brazen, yet to face it all without a quake of knee or, and what is more rare, a tremor of voice; not to forget a syllable; and, in ten minutes, to so cast the spell of a winning personality over his hearers as to evoke a spontaneous outburst of applause, generous from his antagonists, enthusiastic from the nonpartisan. And the medal!

The Professor of English honored our boy by having him at his home to breakfast the following morning, for the double purpose of expressing a genuine appreciation of merit, and of making an impressive bid for his State University attendance next fall.

Aunt Fannie's asthma, with feminine perversity, was at its worst these March nights, and the Squire--fine man that he was--never let his nonimaginative sister know what it cost not to go to Madison with his son-- not to "hear him win the medal." "The trip would cost $10.00; that would get him a fine gold chain to wear his medal on," he ingeniously told her, and thus helped her enjoy her asthma a bit that night, for it was getting a chain for Warren's medal.

The chain and the medal! Was it they that were fated to charm away manhood and nobility and the rich earnest of success? Was it they that were to entice, into this fine promise of fine living, crookedness of thought, unwholesomeness of feeling--dishonorable years?

It was an exuberantly happy victor who returned from the Capitol City with the elaborate gold medal, his name in full conspicuously engraved upon its face--and the youthful society of his school-town was at his feet. Every door was open. So almost without fault was he that few mothers objected to his companionship with their daughters. Yes, here was to be the flaw!--he was soon to find that it was easy for him to have his way with a maid, a dangerous knowledge for a seventeen-year- old boy who had already reached higher social levels than his own home had known, who was much quicker of wit than his almost worshipful father.

It was Eva Martin who had whispered the little prayer-message into his ear that expectant afternoon at the station, and Eva Martin's ear was destined to hear, in turn, whispered pledges of unending devotion, to hear the relentless verdict of unquestioned dishonor.

High school was finished. A successful Freshman year--a Sophomore year that was disappointing to his professors was passed. The fire of his heart was heating many social irons. His earnings, so far, consisted of one gold medal. The savings from the denials at home were about exhausted. The boy had spent as much in the last two years as had been hoped would carry him through college. Fifteen hundred dollars could be raised by remortgaging the farm--it would take this to get him through Law-school, and he was eager to go to Chicago. So a second mortgage was placed. A good deal happened in Chicago which was not written to the Squire nor to Eva. Waring craved being a popular "Hail fellow," and with men, and especially with women, he knew no "No" which would be displeasing. He corresponded with Eva regularly; they would be married some day. He could not have chosen a more superior woman. She lived simply, with her widowed mother, and continued for years to conduct a private kindergarten. She was to save a thousand dollars and he four thousand, then the wedding!

The gray-eyed girl from St. Louis came near saving Eva. Her steel- gray-eyed father's knowledge of human nature alone intervened. It was a chance introduction. She was pretty; she was wealthy. She ran up to Chicago often. Finally the business-like father ran up to Chicago. He invited young Waring to his club for dinner. There were tickets to the "Follies." The younger man let no feature on the stage pass unnoted; the elder remarked every change in the young man's face. There were polite farewells, and a very positive twenty minutes which left the daughter without a question in her mind that further relations with young Waring held most threatening possibilities. Her eyes were not gray without reason, as she proved discreet. There was a bundle of uncomfortably fervid letters which he refused to return.

Warren was shifty with Eva about this affair, and others. He was crooked, too, as the years passed, about his savings. It was impossible to account for certain expenditures, to her. At twenty- eight, she had her thousand dollars in the bank; his supposed four thousand was a bare five hundred, most of which was spent on the gorgeous wedding-trip which he said they both deserved. And shortly after their return to the home, which, instead of being paid for in full, was heavily mortgaged, explanations began which could not explain. Clever as Waring was, his affairs were so involved that Eva could not avoid the suspicion and, soon after, the revelation that her wonderful husband's soul was without honor. It cannot be told, those details of her devoted efforts to "put him right." To forgive anything, everything, she was eager, but he never could come across square, and as the years passed the horror of the uncertain "What next?" enshrouded even her happiest days. Still the husband had ability, and the wife's efforts helped immensely, and there were profitable years. It was odd that, with his declamatory skill, he rarely had a case in court, but proved unusually efficient in developing a collection agency, and gradually represented the Bad Accounts Department of more and more important concerns. At thirty- five he was out of debt. They were living well-- too well it proved, for his nervous health. There must have been a neurotic taint, as expressed in Aunt Fannie's asthma. Early that fall he had his first attack of hay-fever. For years he had been self-indulgent; he always drank when drinks were offered; he used much tobacco and rich food. Athletic he had been; and, advocate of exercise as he was when he gave talks to the boys, he took none himself. So toxins accumulated. He stood this illness poorly. It was the first physical discomfort he had ever known. The family doctor did not help much; patent medicines brought relief. He was pretty hard to live with, these weeks. For a number of years he used the threat of this disorder for a six weeks' trip to Mackinac Island. "Finances" made it possible for the wife and the little boy to spend only two of these weeks with him. During the last four he always managed to keep pace with the fast set. The summer he was forty, the combination of vacation, Mackinac, and fast set did not ward off, in fact did not mitigate, his attacks. Waring returned home "desperate," as he expressed it, and the family doctor succeeded in getting him to a competent Chicago specialist who did some needed nose and throat operations thoroughly and, in spite of careless living, three years of immunity passed. He had become unquestionably a clever handler of bad accounts, and could have made good, had he only been good. A dry, dusty summer, his old enemy, hay-fever-and this time a Chicago "specialist," the kind that advertises in the daily papers, proved his undoing. He gave Waring a spray, potent to relieve and potent to exalt him for hours beyond all touch of lurking apprehension. Bottle after bottle he used; he would not be without it. In a few weeks he realized that he could not be without it. And after the hay-fever days were over he kept using it, furtively now, not only for the exaltation it brought, but as protection from the hellish depression it wrought.

For years Waring's office assistant had been an efficient, devoted, weak woman who had managed well much of the office detail. She now realized that things were not "going straight," that collections made were not being turned over to her, that she was being asked to falsify records. She never could resist his personality, and soon became more adroit than he in juggling figures. Everything went wrong fast. No one suspected cocain--they thought it was whiskey till Eva was forced to tell much to the good old doctor-details revealing her husband's uncouth carelessness of habits, his outbreaks of cruelty to her and the boy, his obvious and shameless lying, his unnatural coarseness of speech. This friend in need spent a bad hour, a hard hour with Waring. Calmness was ineffective, clear reasoning impossible. The accusation of drug-using was vehemently denied, and it was only the doctor's courageous threat to have him arrested and tried on a lunacy charge that broke down the false man's defiance.

Two months of rigid treatment in a sanitarium did much to restore this broken man, and during these weeks the clever office assistant kept his over four-thousand dollar embezzlements from becoming known. Physically and mentally, Waring was restored. The moral sickness was only palliated. When he returned he did not clean house; he swept the dirt into the corners. Frank-facedly he lied to his wife. He met the most pressing of his creditors with a certificate of his illness, and they accepted his notes and promises. He almost crawled out. In so many ways, he was the winning, old "War" Waring again. Gradually, his regime of diet and routine of exercise were replaced by periodic "big eats," little drinks, and many smokes. Then came the warning sneezes and the charlatan's bottle. Irregular living grew apace; the accounts were again manipulated. A Chicago house, which had shown him clemency, became suspicious, and sent a representative who found many collections not reported. A warrant was sworn out, followed by a dozen others after his arrest.

The dear old Squire, now eighty-six, sat beside the brave little wife at the trial. Neither of them thought of forsaking him. As the testimony was given, the old father bowed, mute--as one stricken. The verdict, "Guilty," was returned, and Judge Jefferson had evidently considered carefully his duty. In passing sentence he addressed the criminal: "Warren Waring, the law leaves it with the trial Judge to determine the sentence which shall be passed on you; it may be from five to fifteen years of hard labor in the State Penitentiary. You deserve the full extent of the law's punishment. I have known you from boyhood. Father, wife, God himself, have given you the best they have: an honorable name, a lifetime of devotion, the full ten talents. For these, you have returned dishonor, unchastity and self-indulgent hypocrisy. You have begged extenuation on the basis of nervous ill- health and temporary irresponsibility, both of which you have brought upon yourself by violating the laws of right-living. It is your soul that is sick. You are not fit to live free and equal with righteous men and women. You have had love and mercy-they have failed. Justice will now be given a chance to save you. For the sake of your wife whose noble heart, crushed, pleads for you, I reduce your deserved sentence five years. In respect for your disgraced but honorable father, five additional years are deducted. I pray he may live to see you a free man, chastened. Warren Waring, I sentence you to five years hard labor within the walls of the State Penitentiary."

CHAPTER XVIII

THE BATTLE WITH SELF

The room was bare of furnishings save a cot; no dresser, table, stand, even chair, was there. The windows were of wire glass and guarded by metal screens, the lights were in shielded recesses, the floor was polished but without covering. No pictures, flowers, nor the dainty things which normal women crave were to be seen. On the cot sat a woman, Marie Wentworth, sullen and defiant, a worse than failure, locked in this protected room of a special hospital. Isolated with her caretaker, she was watched day and night-watched to save her from successfully carrying out her determination of self-destruction, a determination which had found expression in more than words, for only the day before-the day of her admission--she had swallowed some cleverly hidden, antiseptic tablets. The trained habits of observation of the skilful nurse had saved her from death. Crafty, vindictive, malicious, reckless, heartless! Her care demanded tireless watching-- hence this room, void of anything by which she could possibly injure herself or others. Nor was she more attractive than her surroundings. Her skin was sallow and unwholesome; yellow-gray rings added dulness to her black eyes. Scrawny of figure, hard and repelling of features, an atmosphere of malevolence seemed to emanate from her presence. She took little note of what was happening, though occasional, furtive glances gave intimation of her knowledge of the nurse's presence. When stimulated to expression there were explosions of violent abuse, directed chiefly against her older sister, explosions punctuated by vicious flashes of profanity which left doubt in no mind of the hatred which rankled-hatred of family, hatred of order and authority, hatred of goodness however expressed, hatred of life and damnations of the hereafter. An unholy picture she was of a demoralized soul in which smoldered and from which flared forth a peace-destroying fire--the rebellion of a depraved body and mind against the moral self. She had been placed in this institution under legal restraint to be treated for morphinism, and, according to her brother, "pure cussedness."

How did it happen? The Wentworths lived well, very well indeed, in a bluegrass county-seat of fair Kentucky. The father was an attorney by profession, a horse-fancier by choice, and for years before Marie's birth relieved the monotony of office duties and race-track pleasures by vivid, gentlemanly "sprees." Marie was only six when his last artery essential to the business of living became properly hardened, and Marie's mother was a widow.

Mrs. Wentworth was to the manor born. She took pride in her home and thoroughly admired the brilliant qualities of her husband. Adorned with old jewels and old lace, she regularly graced her table at the periodic big dinners it was her pride to give. In fact, her pride extended to the planning of three fine meals a day. An unsentimental science suggests that her husband's arteries, as well as her fatal cancer, might have been avoided had chronic proteid intoxication not been the result of her menus. She also took pride in her family and trained the two older children as well as she knew, instilling in them both a loyalty to certain ideals which evolved into morality. But her failing health left Marie much to the care of her sister, and more to the tutelage of her own desires. Unhappily, there was little of beauty in the mother's last months which made any appeal to her child's love, or left much to inspire a twelve-year-old girl's devotion when but memory was left.

When the insurance was collected and all settlements made, the comfortable old home and the jewels sold, each of the three children had five thousand dollars. The brother's success was limited. He invested his all, together with many notes of promise payable to his senior partner, in a dry-goods business, and while he carried most of the details of the establishment, the everlasting interest on his notes, and his wife's love of and demand for fine feathers, kept ends from ever successfully meeting.

The sister, the eldest, was fine. The illness and death of her parents laid grave responsibilities on her young life, and she met them seriously, wholesomely, constructively. She early proved herself capable of large sacrifices. She had finished her college course before her mother's death, and after the home was sold she secured a position in the local woman's college, where she continued to teach and to merit a growing respect for many years. She was not perfect; the Wentworth temper flashed out most inopportunely, and work and pray and sacrifice and resolve as she would, her rule of Marie was unfortunate-flint and steel strike fire. Probably she "school-manned" rather than mothered the child.

But with all environment favorable, Marie would have proven a "proposition." The sporting blood and Bourbon high-balls of the father and the mother's love of the good things of life more than neutralized the latter's Methodism. Marie was a healthy, well-built, lithe lassie, with raven-black hair and eyes which snapped equally with pleasure or with wrath. Impulsive, intense, wilful, tempestuous, bright and possessing capacity, pleasure-loving and ever impatient of restraint, we see in her the highly developed nervous temperament. She feared nothing save the "horrible nightmares" which frequently followed the big dinners-a child who could have been led to Parnassus, but who was driven nearly to Hell! She went through the public schools without conscious effort, but her buxom figure, the rich flush of health, her vivacity, her bearing, were irresistible to the youth of the community, and a series of escapades culminated in her dismissal from college; her indiscretions cost her the respect of the one man she loved. At twenty she had spent two thousand of the five thousand left her, while she and the sister failed to find harmony together. She had little sympathy with her sister's plodding life, but realized the need of preparing herself to earn, so entered a Cincinnati hospital. She had many qualities which made her a valuable student-nurse, with propensities which kept her in hot water. She had completed her second year of training when she was dismissed. The interns could not resist her, nor she them, and only so many midnight lunches on duty can be winked at, even in a hospital needing nurses. For nearly a year she was spasmodically occupied as an experienced nurse. The end of this year found her one thousand dollars poorer, while her heritage was becoming more manifest. In the place of her father's periodic alcoholism, it was periodic headaches. She was thoroughly impatient of personal suffering, or of any hygienic restraint, and so took heavy doses of headache-powders and, if these did not relieve, opiates. By falsifying her record, she succeeded in entering another training- school, a smaller one, in her own state. For a year she was careful- she was anxious to graduate-and developed real cunning in the use of drugs; but dependence upon these steadily undermined her reserve until she was almost daily using something for the "tired feeling" which was now so chronic. Nearly two years had passed before her drug-taking habit was discovered. Prompt dismissal necessarily followed. Her sister was informed, and insisted upon her going to an institution to be cured. Five hundred dollars were spent, and three months of treatment, directed to the withdrawal of her drug, gave no insight into her need for seriously altering her habits of life and feeling, brought no least conception of her defects of character without change of which there could be, for her, no safe living.

During the next ten years her physical and mental deterioration increased apace. Other courses of treatment were taken with no lasting benefit. Her misfortunes seemed to culminate when she voluntarily entered a "drug-cure" institute which was practically a resort for drug-users. There are in every country unworthy places of this kind, where no real effort to cure patients is made. Sufferers with means are kept comfortable by being given drugs whenever they demand them, thus satisfying their consciences that they are being "treated," while vainly waiting till they are sufficiently strong to get entirely off "dope." In such a house of quackery Marie stayed two years. Her remaining fifteen hundred dollars and a thousand of her sister's went for fake treatment. She learned to smoke cigarettes with the young doctor; she played cards, gossiped, ate, slept and was never refused a comforting dose whenever she couldn't "stand it a minute longer." Worse than wasted years these, for even the remnants of her pride faded, and she lived a sordid life of the flesh. The sister, when she finally realized the gravity of the situation, lost all hope whatever for any restoration and, acting under the advice of the old family physician, had her committed to the State Hospital for the Insane as an incurable narco-maniac. Here she was rudely but promptly deprived of all narcotics, nor by any hook nor crook, cunning though she was, could she secure a quieting, solacing grain. The wise superintendent, believing that there was little chance for her true regeneration in the surroundings of even his best wards, advised that she be sent to a hospital where she would receive special care. The sister's funds alone could make this possible, and her genuine worth is shown in her willingness to spend a quarter of her entire savings that Marie might have this chance. Here, thirty-three years old, we found her the day after she had been transferred, the day after she had vainly tried to carry out her vow to end things if she were ever "forced into another treatment."

Throughout the years the primitive self had been pitted against her own soul. She had always rebelled at her misfortunes, though they were largely of her own making. She blamed others for her hardships, and through the intensity of her resentment but made things harder. Not the least expression of her depravity was her hatred for all who had interfered with her wilful desires, particularly the sister, whose sacrifice she ignored, but whom she took a malicious delight in proclaiming to be the one who had forever ruined her chances in life by committing her to an insane asylum. But her delight was malicious, and all that she got out of her hate and maligning was deeper misery. The bitter dregs of twenty years of soulless living were all the cup of life now held for her--all the more bitter because of the finer qualities of her nature. There were possibilities in this highly organized girl which could have led her into an unusual wholeness of living.

Six months passed, months of sullen, dogged resistance-resistance to the returning health which was again rounding her form and glowing her cheeks, resistance to proffered kindnesses of fellow-patients and nurses, resistance to any appeal to pride, honor, ambition, right. Sick of soul, she abjured the interest of the hospital workers, the love of her sister whose weekly letters she left unopened, the wholesome atmosphere of her surroundings, the personal appeal of those whose hearts were heavy with desire to help.

Then the miracle!-for one came who cast out devils. She was not only a nurse, she was one of those divinely human beings who, with a nurse's knowledge and training, attain practical sainthood. She, too, had frequently been repelled in her hours of contact with this unhappy creature, but she believed that under all this unholiness there was a soul. She was a busy, hard-worked nurse, but in time Marie became aware that she was spending part of her limited off-duty hours to minister to her, that she had requested a special assignment of duty which would throw them together. Marie's four years of training made her recognize the rareness of this giving. Curiosity at least was aroused, and she began asking personal questions. An unconscious self-pity impelled her to discuss the grievances of the life of nursing, the unfairness common in training-schools, the injustices of long hours and inadequate appreciation, with scores of other quarrels which she had with life. Each of these was met squarely by her nurse-friend, who, free from platitudes and cant, ever saw the ideal above it all, who, loving her profession and loving humanity and promised to a life of service, gently, beautifully, firmly stood by her principles. For three months they were in daily contact--three thankless months for the nurse, three months of cunning, evil-minded, suspicious testing by the patient. Finally the very goodness of her friend seemed intolerable, and a paroxysm of rage and resentment broke loose, in which she cursed and abused her helper beyond sufferance. The nurse suddenly grasped the unhappy woman's arms to shake some sense of decency into her warped nature, one would have thought, but in truth that eye might meet eye, and in this look the rare love, which can persist through such provocation, awakened a soul. That look was at once the revelation of the worth of the one and the worthlessness of the other. A flood of tears drowned, it would seem forever, the evil which was cursing. In a day, in an hour, the change was wrought, that miraculous change which enters every life when the soul comes into its own.

There were months in which the battle of self ebbed and flowed, but never did defeat seem again imminent, and the final victory was found in a high resolve which took her back home a quiet, subdued woman, forgetful of self in her sense of debt to the sister whose goodness she had never before admitted. For years they lived together, she keeping the simple home and keeping it well, saving, industrious, devoted, even loving. She has largely avoided publicity, though always ready to nurse in emergencies. Nobly she is expiating the past, and has long since worthily won the "well-done" of her moral self.

CHAPTER XIX

THE SUFFERING OF SELF-PITY

Alac MacReady was not much of an oarsman. Big and strong, and heretofore so successful that his large self-confidence had never been badly jolted, he was quite at a disadvantage, this June afternoon, as he attempted to row pretty Annette Neil across the head of the lake to where she said the fishing was good. Twice already he had splashed her dainty, starched frock, ironed, he knew, in the highest perfection of the art, by her own active, shapely, brown hands. And each awkward splashing had been followed by flashing glances which shriveled self- esteem even as they fascinated. They had planned to spend the sunset hour fishing, then land in time to meet the crowd and be driven on to Border City to a neighboring dance, and all come back to Geneva together.

Alac's rural North-England training had developed in him many qualifications of worth but, among these, boating was not one. Had he told the truth when this little trip was planned, he would have admitted that he had never rowed a boat a half-mile in his life. Annette could do it tip-top; why not he? But things were unquestionably perverse. The boat wouldn't go in a straight line- in fact, it didn't go very fast anyway. The black eyes before him framed by that impudently beautiful face, so pert, so naive, so understandingly aware-- so "damned handsome" he said to himself, prodded him to redoubled effort. He was swinging his two hundred pounds lustily, unevenly--an unusually vicious jerk, and snap went the old oar! Off the seat he tumbled, and, with land-lubber's luck, unshipped the other oar and away it floated, and a mile from land, they drifted.

Alac MacReady was Scotch-English. The family had executed a number of important contracts for the British government; one of these had brought two of the boys to Canada. With their family backing, they had undertaken some constructive work in northern New York, and, at this time, were building a railroad which passed through Geneva. Alac had been in the neighborhood for two months supervising operations. He was striking in appearance--a florid-faced' blonde, brusque in business, quite jovial socially, and cracking--full of the conceit of youth, wealth and station. So far, life had, in practically nothing, refused his bidding.

Annette Neil's father kept a small store, Annette did much of the clerking. She was unquestionably the prettiest girl in Geneva; indeed she was as pretty as girls are made. With all her small-town limitations she was bright as a pin, and as sharp; fine of instinct and, withal, coy as a coquette. The first time Alac addressed her it was as a shop-keeper. Something she said kept turning over in his brain and he realized next morning, as he was shaving, that her reply had been impertinent. Piqued, he returned the day after to make another purchase, and made the greater mistake of being patronizing. Mr. Alac MacReady discovered, without any prolonged period of rumination, that he had a bee in his bonnet, and left the little shop semispeechless and irate. He was not satisfied to leave the honors with this "snip of an American girl," and evolved a plan of verbal assault which was to bring the provincial upstart to her senses, only to discover that she had a dozen defenses for each attack, and to find himself, for two consecutive, disconcerting minutes, wondering if perchance he might be a "boob." With each visit--and they were almost daily and many of them made in the face of strong, contrary resolution--he felt the distinction in their stations disappearing. He later found himself calling on Annette's mother, and, stiffly at first, later humbly asking for the company of the bewitching girl, who, coy witch that she was, steadfastly refused to be "company" even when her mother said she might. This trip across the lake was the first real concession the little minx had made-and how "bloomingly" he "messed it up"! He was not used to the water, and, oarless, became "panicky." A pair of ridiculing eyes caused him to break off his second bellow for help, in its midst.

The little boat drifted slowly. The June breeze was not strong. The sun slipped behind radiant clouds, clouds which shifted and softened, and tinted and toned through the pastels into the neutrals. Gently they were nearing the shore when the great, golden moon rose in the east, and soon brightening, shimmered the lake with countless, dancing splotches of silver. The water lapped with ceaseless, dainty caresses the sides of the boat. Some mother-bird nestling near the water's edge crooned her good-night message to her mate. A halo surrounded and softened the white face so near and, as part of the evening symphony, two dark eyes rested upon his face, deeply luminous. There are different stories of what he said. He admitted he was never so awkward. But they missed their companions, and the dance, and walked all the way 'round the head of the lake, home, this proud son of near- nobility doing obeisance to his untutored queen. So Alac and Annette married. They traveled far, first to Canada, then to England. Annette's sheer beauty and remarkable taste in the use of Alac's prodigal gifts of clothing and jewels carried the badly disturbed and certainly unfavorably prejudiced MacReady family by assault. Ten years they lived in the big Northumberland home. A boy and a girl came, both blondes like their father. The MacReady boys were not meeting the same success in their contracting ventures for which two former generations had been noted. And, after their father's death, one particularly disastrous contract quite reduced the family's financial standing and consequent importance. The three brothers could not agree as to which was to blame, so Alac and his family returned to America and located in Rochester. Their few thousands Alac invested in a small manufacturing concern which never prospered sufficiently to maintain him in his life-long habits of good living. Unhappily, too, strong as Alac was in many ways, his one weakness grew. Three or four times a year he would make trips to Toronto or New York, drink gloriously, spend hundreds of dollars, and return home meek and dutiful, almost praying Annette not to say what he knew was in her mind. Of the two children, little Alac multiplied his father's weaknesses by an unhappily large factor. He never amounted to much, developing little but small bombast. Charlotte was the child, dutiful, studious, rather serious perhaps, but very conscientious. Her features were those of neither father nor mother, but peculiarly delicate, strikingly refined. When she was fifteen her father was found dead, one morning, in an obscure hotel in the Middle West. He had neglected his insurance premiums. The resourceful little widow went to work at once. The products of her needle were exquisite. She sold some of the handsome old furniture and, during the next five years, most of her jewels went to keep the children in school. She had given absolutely to her husband and to her home, and through the years to come her cheer was never bedimmed save when the husband was mentioned. Charlotte became more attractive. She was slender, fair--the English type was apparent; she was a distinct contrast to her highly colored, brunette mother, who, however, might have been but an older sister, she had so preserved her youth. Charlotte was periodically morbid, a transmuted heritage. The financial need directed her training into practical lines; she studied stenography and was fortunate in securing a position in the office of John Evanson, the energetic senior member of a growing leather-manufacturing firm. There was something poetically appealing to this busy man in the quiet, sometimes sad-faced, fine- faced, competent woman, which gradually created in him a hungering sense of need-and he called one night. He afterwards said if he hadn't married Charlotte, he would have married her mother, who, to tell the truth, put what sparkle there was into the courtship.

Charlotte's cup of happiness should have been overflowing when she moved into the handsome, big house. Her mother was to live with them, and such a mother-in-law would be a welcome asset to any home. Mr. Evanson gave Alac Junior the only good position he ever had--a position which he never filled to any one's satisfaction but his own. For two years Charlotte's virtues were expressed in quiet, almost thoughtful home-devotion, entertainment of poor relatives, and church- work. John Evanson was simple and rational in his tastes. In business he was enterprising and a keen fighter of competition. He cleverly managed his interests, which had grown through years of steadfast attention. He was nearly forty when he married, and his new home was to him a haven. The mother adapted herself superbly and was a real joy in the household through her wit and daintiness and ingenious thoughtfulness.

Charlotte was not well for several months before the birth of the much-wished-for baby, which unhappily never breathed. A sharp illness which lingered was followed by eight miserable months, then an operation, and the surgeon pronounced her well-but she could not believe she was. Two years of rather unassuming semi-invalidism passed. She made few complaints; she was evidently repressing expression of the recurring symptoms of her discomfort. But since her baby's death she had recovered little ability for effort. She tired quickly. She was living a life of quiet, sheltered, almost luxurious inadequacy. Dr. Corning was puzzled. Mrs. Evanson had appealed to his professional pride and sympathetic nature strongly. Was there something obscure, a lurking condition which he had overlooked? He would have his work reviewed by the celebrated New York internist. Nothing was found which resulted helpfully. Mrs. MacReady was patient. Her innate good judgment withheld discussion of details with her unhappy daughter. She believed Charlotte to be secretly mourning for the little one who had not lived. She spent hours with her son-in-law in anxious conference. What could get her poor child out of this almost apathy? She looked so well; she had never weighed so much; but twice she had been found looking over the baby's things. Was her sorrow eating away at her heart? Hadn't he noticed that for months she left the room when her father or the baby was mentioned! And hadn't he noticed the marks of tears when she came back? The husband had never loved his wife more; he pitied her; he yearned to share the burden which she did not mention. He watched the change in her moods and brought something new each day to please, divert, to interest-books and flowers, periodicals, clothing, jewelry. Pets proved tiresome. She wearied soon on every attempted trip. Concerts and the theater, and music in the home, all made her "nervous."

Mrs. MacReady firmly believed the trouble was a haunting spirit of unsatisfied mother-love, and suggested bringing a child into the home. This plan did arouse new interest. Months were spent in making the selection. Scores of points must be satisfactorily fulfilled, or the plan would prove but a bitter disappointment. At last, a nine-months- old girl-baby was discovered who promised to resemble her foster- mother, and who had a "respectable heritage 'way back on both sides." It seemed most fortunate for both the little orphan and the hungering woman-this adoption. Charlotte spent much time in getting the little one outfitted and settled. The child brought new problems, such as worthy nursemaids, sleep-hours and safe feeding-and Charlotte was better.

Mrs. MacReady had not been looking well. For months she had been slowly losing weight, although there had been not a syllable of complaint. Mr. Evanson finally insisted-the examination revealed an incurable condition--presto! Charlotte was prostrated. The trained nurse, secured for the mother, spent most of her time attending the multiplying needs of the daughter, whose apprehension grew until she began sending for her husband during his office-hours, fearing that her mother was worse; or because she looked as if she might have one of the hemorrhages the doctor feared, or to discuss what they would do when her mother died. The months dragged on. The splendid mother radiated cheer to the last. Then began the reign of terror. Stimulants and sedatives seemed necessary to protect Charlotte from "collapse." For a month, Mr. Evanson did not go near the office; for years, he was subject to calls by day, was disturbed mercilessly at night. No nurse could fill his place. It seemed chiefly the sick woman's "heart." Dr. Corning was too frank-Charlotte insisted he did not "understand." Dr. Winton was "sympathetic." He was physician for many society women. He was an adept in providing understanding and comfort. He never advised "dangerous operations or nasty mixtures," and was no fanatic on diet and exercise.

When Charlotte married, she was "lily-fair," and weighed one hundred and sixteen. Five years after her mother's death she was florid, vapid, and weighed one hundred and sixty-eight miserable pounds. She ran the gamut of nervous ailments: disturbances of circulation, digestion, breathing, eating, sleeping, antagonism to draughts and noises, and a special antipathy to the odor from the exhaust of motor- cars. This last made her faint, and of her fainting attacks pages might be written. The home of John Evanson was now a dreary place. It was a household subsidized to the whims of a self-pitying woman. Her loss of father, baby and mother had "wrecked her life." Husband, child, nurse, servants, were all under the blight of her enslaving self-commiseration. For years all church and social activities were unattempted. Relatives and friends could not be entertained, for every one's attention was demanded to meet the varying possible emergencies of symptoms and to keep her mind from dwelling on her losses and the wretchedness of her fate.

Mr. Evanson's business interests were neglected. His devotion to his morbid, now thoroughly selfish wife lost him big opportunities. His nerves, too, suffered from the unceasing strain. Serious-minded, nonimaginative, honest, it never occurred to him that the illness of his "poor afflicted wife" was an illness of the soul only. The adopted daughter was surrounded by an atmosphere of unnatural repression, an atmosphere charged with false sympathy and unwholesome concessions to the selfish weaknesses of her foster-mother. Dr. Winton advised many comfortable and diverting variations in treatment, but life in the Evanson home became increasingly distorted. At last John realized he was losing out badly-he must have a change. Through some subconscious inspiration he took Dr. Winton with him. They spent two weeks hunting and fishing in the Maine woods. John sought to get in touch with the man behind the doctor. The doctor soon realized the manliness of his companion. They were resting after a taxing portage, both feeling the fine exhilaration of perfect physical relaxation after productive physical weariness. The two men were pretty close. Shop had not been mentioned during the two weeks.

"Doctor, tell me about my wife, just as though she were a sister."

The doctor mused several minutes. "It is not pleasant... it is not easy to tell... you won't want to hear it. You probably will not accept what I have to say... you may resent it."

"Tell me straight; you know how vitally I and my household need to understand the truth."

Gravely the physician spoke--as friend to friend: "Your wife has leprosy!--not the physical form, but the kind that anesthetizes, ulcerates, deforms the soul--the leprosy of self-pity. It began with her father's death. It has eaten deeper and deeper, fed by the unselfishness of her mother and of yourself, unchecked by the soothing salves applied by doctors like me. I early recognized that she would not pay the price of radical cure--the price of effortful living. Her understanding soul has degenerated--something vital to Christ-like living is, I believe, lost. She believes her undiseased body to be ill. Her reason is distorted by her disease-obsessions; her will has been pampered into a selfish caricature. She has accepted the false counsel of her selfishness so long that she is attracted by error, and repelled by truth. I see relief for her only through the culminating self-deception that disease does not exist. If this error is accepted by her, she will become as fanatically superior to her wretched sensations as she is now subservient to them. In other words, she is a worse than useless woman whom Christian Science may transform. She is emotionally sick. Christian Science appeals to the emotional life; it is not concerned with reason-no more is she. It negates physical illness and thus might replace her morbid, hopeless, selfish sufferings with years of applied, wholesome cheer and faith."

Some details were discussed. A fine personality, a woman who devoutly accepted the teachings of Mrs. Eddy, who would have been an example of selfless living, regardless of details of religious faith, was interested in poor Charlotte. Progress was slow at first. Then the leaven began to work. One day the expressman moved a big box from the Evanson home to a local hospital. It contained the paraphernalia of a one-time invalid. One plastic nurse lost a chronic case. To-day in the Evanson household, all discussions of illness are under the ban. The home is no longer a private infirmary, but breathes a bit of the after-glow of cheer which should linger long after the passing of one so worthy and radiant as Annette--the mother beautiful in body and spirit.

CHAPTER XX

THE SLAVE OF CONSCIENCE

In the following life-story, our sympathies are strongly drawn to the conscientious woman who gave so many years of uncomplaining service--a giving which should have brought its daily reward of satisfaction; yet she sorrowed through her youth because she lacked the charity that "suffereth long and is kind," finding which, her problem was met.

The never too attractive Yarnell home was in a mess. Irene, the eight- year-old child, seemed seriously ill. The doctor had said, the night before, that they might have to operate if the pain in her side didn't get better; and the little girl prayed that they would, and prayed specially that she would die while they were doing it. She didn't want to live. She wanted to go rather than to stay forever with the new mother her father had brought home last month. Big Sister wouldn't stay; she ran away the second week and married Tim Shelby, and had a good home now with Tim's people--even though her father hadn't spoken to the Shelbys for years. Aunt Erne had gone too, dear Aunt Erne, her mother's sister, who had been mother to her ever since her real mother died--just after she was born--that precious mother, who, Aunt Effie used to tell her, had died happy that her little girl might live. Aunt Effie had always taught her a beautiful love, and every night she said a beautiful prayer for the mother she had never seen. Aunt Effie tried to stay, too, but couldn't. She left the same day the new mother asked father, before them all, how he was ever going to keep up with all the expenses of so many and give a tenth of his salary to the church.

The very night her aunt went away, the step-mother had told Irene that it was wicked to "do up" her hair in curl-papers, and when she begged her, "Just this once," because she had a "piece to speak" in school next day, and cried in her disappointment, her stepmother had shaken her so hard that something seemed to tear loose in her side. Irene had never hated any one before--and it was wicked to hate; and so she was praying her real mother to come and take her before she became a sinner. But in spite of her prayers, she shrank when her stepmother came near and chilled whenever touched by her. She couldn't eat the food she brought, and every time she thought of her, the pain was worse. Both her father and his new wife seemed so strange. She felt like some stray, hurt animal, not loved by any one.

The new Mrs. Yarnell had been a maiden-lady many years. During her spinsterhood she had given herself without stint to the activities of her small church, a church belonging to an obscure denomination which teaches that holiness is nigh upon us; that if we but supplement conversion by a second act of grace, sanctification here and forevermore is ours. Hers was not an easy disposition to live with. She had ably held her own through years of bickerings and wordy contentions with an overworked, irritable mother. She gave little love. She received little. But her underdeveloped, souring heart instinctively craved some drops of sweetness. So, when she listened to the fervid exhorter, revealing the new highway to heaven, that glorious way where the good Lord carries all our burdens, if we will just cast them upon Him, a great light illumined her soul. Why a weary life of strife and misunderstanding? She would give herself without reserve, and even in the giving she could feel her burden roll away. In a flash it seemed, life had changed. She was now the Lord's--mind, soul and body. He directed; she followed. He could not lead her wrong, and, as all her impulses and desires were now divine, she could do no wrong. She could think no wrong. Having given all, she was now saved to the uttermost. Misunderstood she must be, of course, by those who knew not the holy leadings of her sanctified soul. Serenely, supremely, she lived. Her old biting temper was now righteous indignation. Her dislike for household work was only an evidence that, like beautiful Mary, she had chosen the better part. What her mother had always called obstinacy and perversity were now stead-fastness in the Lord. Oddly, her tart, sarcastic, even flaying tongue was not softened by any gentleness of divine inspiration. Incidentally, the Lord had given her a plump figure, and a knack of apparel which had long appealed to Widower Yarnell's eye. And the Lord approved; in truth He said "Yes!" so audibly that Miss Spinster hesitated hut one maidenly minute.

Mrs. Yarnell's sanctification washed dishes, kept house, and nursed lonely, sick, little children most inefficiently. So, after Aunt Effie and Big Sister, both willing workers, left, the new bride found unforeseen difficulties in following the Lord's leadings, which seemed to call to real back-and-muscle taxing effort for other people--such was for the world of Marthas. So things in the Yarnell household got in a mess.

It seemed hard for Irene to recover. But her returning strength found early tonic in the house-work which was left for her to do. The new mother's church activities occupied so much of her time that little was left for any but unavoidable essentials. Irene became a fine little worker, and should have had all the honors and happiness due the model child. Neat, rapid, effective, an excellent student, she developed physically strong, the possessor of that rare and attractive glow of health, into a thoroughly wholesome looking young woman. Deep within, however, she had not known peace since the day Aunt Effie left. For years she had fought smoldering resentment and an embittering sense of injustice, until at fourteen the deeper depths were stirred by a slow but irresistible religious awakening. Her stepmother's church was on the opposite side of town, too far for them both to attend. Her own mother's church was in the neighborhood, and throughout the years she had usually been able to attend Sunday-school there and be home again in time to get dinner. Her young understanding had long been in a turmoil as to what religion and right are. Aunt Effie had taught gentleness of conduct and charity of speech, and forgetfulness of self in service. Mrs. Yarnell constantly proclaimed that, until the Lord entered her heart to absolutely sanctify it, she was certain to be miserable, unless she became a hopelessly hardened sinner.

Unhappy the child surely was. Her conscience was a sensitive one; it seemed ever to chide, and often to condemn. No matter how faithfully she followed duty, her failure to receive that wonder-working "second blessing" left her feeling as an unworthy one outside of the fold. Then, when she neglected, even for an hour, her household duties or school-work for church-socials or class-picnics, her conscience, and usually her step-mother, pounced upon her mercilessly. At early fourteen, she was feeling the chilling shadows of a morbid conscience. Her stepmother was away for two weeks attending a denominational conference, and it seemed to Irene that she had more time than usual; so she talked her perplexities over with the pastor of her mother's church. A good man he was, but far from being an expert physician of the soul. He did not seem to sense her deeper problem-the one daily hurting her sensitive spirit, but asked a number of questions, her answers to which convinced him that she was entirely ready to join the church, which he definitely advised her to do, believing thereby she would find the peace she sought. So without delay, even before her stepmother's return, and without consulting her, she followed the minister's advice. Unhappily, her business-burdened father had no special interest in the welfare of any one's soul. Mrs. Yarnell henceforth treated Irene as a religious inferior. High school brought more work and little play. The unsuccessful father died with bad arteries when Irene was eighteen. He left little beside the mortgaged place; so Irene took up bookkeeping, and before she was twenty had a bank-position which, through her ability and merit and trustworthy conscientiousness, she has held through the years and the vicissitudes, supporting herself and her stepmother. Irene's play days had been rare. Her conscience was a grim-visaged angel whose flaming sword she ever saw barring each path to pleasure.

The president of her bank was also an elder in her church. His mind was pretty well filled with business, still he took occasional thought for his employees, and the summer Irene was twenty-three, he asked her how she would spend her two vacation weeks. "No," she was not going to leave Wheeling. "Yes," it was hot, but she had much sewing to do, and if she could save for two years more, the mortgage would be paid. The banker noticed, even as they talked, the slight tremor of fingers and lips which bespeaks tension; and that not a little of her appearance of reserve and strength had slipped away through the grind of the years.

Three delegates were to be sent to the Chautauqua Assembly for a two weeks' special conference, and somehow it turned out that, with those of Mrs. Crumb, the pastor's wife, and Matthew Reynolds, a theologic student the church was helping educate, Irene Tarnell's name was read. Two weeks at Chautauqua, her railway-fare paid both ways!-a score of the best people of the church assuring her that it was her duty-and an envelope with the banker's personal check for twenty dollars, endorsed "for incidentals as delegate"! Thus Irene set forth on her first foreign mission, her first trip out into this big, busy world, about which she had, wrongfully, of course, wasted a few minutes now and then in dreaming. Who could have been more companionable than Matthew, or who more thoughtful and self-eliminating than Mrs. Crumb whose thrifty, matronly heart early sensed the promise and wisdom-and excitement, too, of a romance en route. And dear Mrs. Crumb was deft, and Matthew supremely susceptible, and Irene-she was in the clouds! How like a story-book, the kind that ends happily, it would have worked out, if alas! Matthew had not been quite so susceptible. There was a Pittsburgh girl who had the advantage of prior association and, unfortunately, the young student's pledge of eternal devotion. Still, Irene was a mighty good-looking girl; in fact, Matthew admitted, the third day of their trip, when her fine color began to flash back, that she was better looking than his promised, and so refreshingly free from worldly-mindedness. Mrs. Crumb did not know of Matthew's entanglements, while the devotion of his attentions, a certain lighting of his eyes, and gentleness of speech and demeanor convinced her that all she wished was going very well. So convinced was she that she made bold, early the second week, to express her belief in Irene's almost unequaled qualifications for a minister's wife, to which dutiful Matthew gave unreserved assent.

Nothing of importance was scheduled for Wednesday afternoon, and Mrs. Crumb showed that she was not lacking in an understanding of young folks' human nature when she planned the little excursion which was to offer ample opportunity for the consummation she believed so impending. They had all taken some tramps together. She was not quite equal, she said, to the walk around to Mayfield, but it would make a fine afternoon trip for the young folks. She would go down on the steamer, and they could all come back and enjoy the refreshing, evening water-trip together.

Matthew had certainly been attentive, giving an attention which Irene had never before received. For days she had been happy, the first joy- days she had known since she was eight. The very near future loomed large with intoxicating promise. Mrs. Crumb had talked to her, also, of Matthew, and of his fine record at college, and of his gentle nature. The early afternoon was hot; they walked slowly; they loitered when they came to shade. Then out of the west came booming black clouds, and they were caught in a mid-summer thunderstorm. He helped her as they ran for shelter, but, almost blinded by the pelting rain, she tripped and fell awkwardly, twisting her ankle cruelly. She probably fainted. Matthew was frightened, and in his helplessness lost his head. She was roused by him chafing her hands, and his importunate "Dear Irene," bundled stunned senses, soaked, chilling apparel and stabbing ankle into one unutterable confusion of unspeakable joy. And "devil-inspired fool" that she was, she reached up, drew his tense face, so near, against hers, and "hateful bliss," it stayed there a full minute. Then life went black, for he tore himself away, almost savagely putting her arm aside. "It is wrong; you have made me sin!"

"It is wrong; you have made me sin!" were burned in loathsome black across the face of her conscience, accusing cruelly, unendingly accusing. Tears passed-those years that drag, and she never knew of the girl in Pittsburgh. She did not know other than that she had transgressed and tempted a fine, good man; that she had tempted him from the sanctity of great religious purpose-and her branded, sick conscience proved itself a poison to mind and body.

Dazed, the hurt woman returned to the loveless home. Mechanically, for months, her hands made that home comfortable and toiled on at the bank. We wonder how the break could have been held back so long, in one so sensitive. The staunch body and well-trained mind must have carried her on through mere momentum. But it had to come. Self- condemnation and self-depreciation gave birth to false self- accusation. She began to question the worth of all she did. Repeatedly she must add and re-add a column of figures; even the evidence of the adding-machine had to be proven. She wakened at night questioning the correctness of her entries, and her work became slow and inaccurate. All she did, physically and mentally, became a dread. The very act of walking to and from the bank seemed to drain her waning strength. She refused a vacation suggested by her employer, who gradually became genuinely concerned about her health. He knew but little of the affair at Chautauqua. Mrs. Crumb was too good a woman to let drop any hint of what she may have surmised; she actually knew only of the storm and sprained ankle.

One morning Mrs. Yarnell called a neighboring doctor. She couldn't waken Irene. It was found that her sleep had become so poor that she had bought some powders from the druggist. Never having taken medicine, she was easily influenced, and the ordinary dose left her confused for twenty-four hours. Two weeks' rest at home, if one could rest in Mrs. Yarnell's company, found the girl no stronger. The banker and the doctor had a conference. She must be gotten away from home. The banker had a doctor-friend, a man whose means made it unnecessary for him to give his years of strength to the unceasing demands of a general practice. He had long been keenly interested in the complicated and growing problem of nervousness. He owned a beautiful place down the Ohio River where, for years, he had been taking into his home a few deserving, nervous invalids. He had learned to enter into their lives with a specialist's skill-with a father's understanding. Thus he gave largely--to some it would seem, of his substance, but the true giving was his discerning, constructive comprehension of human problems. Into this atmosphere, God and the banker sent Irene.

For nearly twenty years this oversensitive girl had known few hours of understanding and sympathy. For a week or two she merely rested; then one evening, it seemed precipitate, but some way it was as easy as anything she had ever done, she told the story we have heard. There, revealed, was the defect of a life, a problem to be worked out by the analytic student of mankind. Was it to introduce a little saving recklessness, the redeeming truth of honesty and justice to self, or the neutralizing of self-negation by the acceptance of merited worth! Even through our weaknesses are we sometimes healed. If any reason existed which could merit one self-accusing thought, the doctor found it when he uncovered the resentment which had never healed toward the usurping stepmother--"a woman who had proved her limitations and should be mercifully judged thereby," he told Irene.

"Yes," the doctor said, "you have missed the 'second blessing'; you have missed a thousand blessings because the generosity of your years of fine doing were lacking in the gentleness of feeling which Aunt Effie taught you, and which made your mother so beloved. Lacking this, even in the fulness of your much giving, you have failed. You have been seeking the true religion. Your mother had it-the kind that lightens the dead heaviness and puts heaven's color into the dull, dark hours at home. Herein, only, have you fallen short."

The doctor knew men, and he was able to show her how utterly innocent she was of the slightest hint of wrong in her relations with Matthew, how impossible that her spontaneous act could have wrought a second's harm to any good man. There was much more said helpfully, but the most good, unquestionably, came from the unspoken influence of the thoughtful personal consideration and discerning kindness of this scientific lover of his kind. Three months Irene spent with them, the doctor and his equally good wife; she returned home radiant.

The years pass. During the Great War, when trained men were scarce, our restituted woman acted as cashier and drew almost a cashier's salary. The mortgage is paid. Two women live in the little house. The older is very religious. She still attends many church services; she dutifully gives her tenth to the cause, and, in and out of season, proclaims her way as the perfect road to the heights beyond. Old and practically unchangeable, she is not lovable and she never has been, but near-by tenderness has softened some of her self-satisfied asperities. Still radiant is the younger woman-the righteous woman whose righteousness has put unfailing cheer in service most of us would call "fierce," a righteousness which has learned to be charitably blind where most of us would see and resent, a righteousness which has brought abiding happiness to a life that had long suffered, a slave to its conscience. Cleverness and wealth-having not charity-have sought such happiness in vain through the ages.

CHAPTER XXI

CATASTROPHE CREATING CHARACTER

Grandfather Scott was a blacksmith. He was much more-a natural amateur mechanic-the only man in those early days in the little town of Warren, who could successfully tinker sewing-machines, repair clocks, or make a new casting for a broken Franklin heater. He was a hale, ruddy man who lived, worked and died with much peace. There were girls, but David was the only boy, and a lusty youth he was. The absence of brothers, or possibly an excess of sisters, gave him, both as youth and young man, much more liberty of action and right of way than was good for his soul. At any rate, he early developed a steadfastness which, throughout his life, stood for both strength of purpose and hard-headed, sometimes hard-hearted wilfulness. His father had dreamed a dream: his smithy was to grow into a shop, and later the shop was to become a factory where a hundred men would do his bidding and supply the country with products of his inventive genius. But so far as his own life was to realize, it remained a dream. The shop was never built; the genius failed to invent. But his son, David! Yes, he would have the schooling and advantages that the father had not known. And so it was: at thirty, David Scott had been well educated in mechanics; at forty, he had made improvements on the sewing-machine, which gave him valuable patents; at fifty, his factory employed ten times the number his father had visioned. Thus was fulfilled the dream of the ancestor.

Business success was large for Mr. David Scott. But what of his success as a father? He married at twenty-eight, a handsome woman whose pride in appearance stood out through the years and influenced the training given her three children. Little David, or "Dave," as he was early called in distinction to his father, was petted by his mother and, in spite of evidences to the contrary, was his father's pride. The family moved to Cleveland when Dave was a little fellow. His father would not be cramped, so, with what proved to be rare foresight, bought part of an old farm on Mayfield Heights. Both here and at

Granddad's, where Dave was sent each summer, there was ample out-of-doors, and the lad grew sturdy of limb. With a flaming shock of curling, copper hair, his eyes deepest blue, and skin as fair as a girl's, he was a boy for mother, teachers and later for maidens to spoil. But an attractive personality, an inherent fineness never left him while he was conscious, and seldom when he was irresponsible.

Dave's mother was proud, proud of her successful husband, of the mansion and estate of which she was the envied mistress, proud of her handsome self and handsome daughters, and specially proud of Dave, the brightest and handsomest of them all. It is a pity that she who so fully enjoyed the pleasures of wealth, and of wealth-shielded motherhood, might not have lived to drink to her full of the joys she loved. Pride, insufficient clothing, wealth, inadequate exercise, exposure in a raw, March bluster, defective personal resistance, pneumonia!--and in a week, the life was gone.

Dave was only fourteen, but, in face of his spoiling, was ready for St. Paul's, where he was sent the next fall. He was bright-even brilliant in his prep school work. Mathematics, the sciences and history seemed almost play for him, while in languages, and especially in English, he did an unusual amount of "not required" work.

Dave made his father his hero, and for many years was instant in doing his will. Had the older man taken serious thought of his son's personality and entered into the boy's developmental needs with his wonted intelligence and thoroughness, the two could have grown into a closeness which would have made the Scott name one to be reckoned with in the manufacturing world.

The father's business was growing even beyond his own dreams, and he found little time to give his boy, whom, in fact, he saw but rarely, save at Christmas holidays. So it happened that Dave was more deeply influenced by his mother's love for the beautiful than by machine-shop realities; and the aesthetic developed in him to the exclusion of the father's practical life.

For many years wine had been served at the family dinners. Mr. Scott drank only at home, and then never more than two small glasses. He had no respect for the man who overindulged any weakness. He little thought his own blood could be different than he. This father was a man of exceptional energy who had wrought miracles financially, and was, without question, master in his thoroughly organized factory. He dominated his surroundings. Where he willed to lead--whether in business circles, in the vestry, in his own home--the strength of his intellect, the force of his purpose and his quiet but tangible assertiveness were felt. He had never been balked in any determined course of action.

When Dave went East to school, he possessed physique and health which should have made athletics a desire and a joy. But on both the baseball and football squads were a few fellows not choice in their use of English. In fact, even at this excellent church-school, these exceptions did considerable "cussing." Dave's mother and sisters were fastidious, and Dave found himself, even at fourteen, resenting coarseness. He, therefore, chose the "nice fellows" as associates, and made friends to his liking in books. We must not think of him as "prissy" or snobbish, but he distinctly disliked crudity however expressed, and this dislike grew and was strengthened by his increasing devotion to the aesthetic. Otherwise, Dave's prep school years were those of an unusually fine fellow, whose mind promised both brilliance and strength. Sadly, during these vital years, Dave had no mature counselor; no strong character was sufficiently close to sense his needs and court his confidence. So some of the proclivities of his early home influence persisted and developed, which normally should have been displaced by others standing for oncoming manhood.

College life, unfortunately, but increased his opportunities to indulge his weaknesses, and his three years at Yale found him a dependable member of a refined fast-set. With his unusual mind--giving no time to athletics--there were many idle hours at his disposal. He now discovered that he liked cigarettes which his father held in supreme contempt, while, from time to time, a quiet wine-supper with a select few, where spirits blended so finely when mellowed by champagne, stood for the acme of social pleasure. Dave could not carry much liquor and mellowed early, and rather soon slipped quietly under the table, to be told the next day most of the snappy toasts and stories the other fellows had contributed to the occasion. These entertainments soon forced Dave to overdraw his allowance. A business- like letter asking explanations came from his father, and this was followed by a peremptory command that he live within his already "ample remittance." Father and son had never been companions, and here the boy's devotion deserted, and a growing estrangement began. Dave, knowing his father's wealth, resented his lack of liberality, and he knew him too well to protest. For three months he heeded parental injunction; then a trip to New York to grand opera. Entertainment accepted must be returned. Another wine-supper, paid for by a draft on his father-and family warfare was on! The draft was paid-the family credit must not be questioned, but a house was divided against itself, and the letter David sent Dave left a trail of blue smoke. It left also a reckless, rebellious son.

Adelaide Foster's grandfather was wealthy. Her mother had suited her own taste-not her parents'-when she married attractive Fred Foster. The grandfather dallied too often with the "bucket-shop" before he forgave his foolish child, and when he came to his better paternal self, he hadn't much to leave his little granddaughter. But Adelaide made much of her little, and spent two very developing years at Barnard.

Dave and Adelaide met on terms artistic which were most satisfying to them both. Dave had made good junior marks in spite of his inoffensive sprees and conflicts with his father. He was in many ways Adelaide's superior, but she gave him a large companionship in things beautiful, and worshiped at his feet in questions profound. His father had ignored, or failed to notice, Dave's references to the young lady-so there was a little wedding-ceremony with four witnesses, an almost impulsive wedding. The elder Scott was not expecting this flank- movement, but family pride again helped Dave out, and a liberal check followed the stiff telegram of "best wishes."

Six months the young folks spent abroad. The beautiful in nature and art which Europe offered blended into their honeymoon. The last wedding-gift dollar had been spent when they returned to East Best, the paternal mansion in Cleveland. Two evenings later Mr. Scott called his son into the library. It was time to reassert his sovereignty. This, too, was business; so it was curt and direct. "Well, sir, I trust you have sown your wild oats. You have married. It is high time you settled down. I shall give you and Adelaide a home with us, or, if you prefer to live elsewhere, one hundred dollars a month for living expenses. This, mark you, is my gift to her. You don't earn a cent of it. You will have to start in the business at the bottom. You may choose the shops or the office. You will be paid what you earn. I hope you will make good. You are capable. Good-night."

Dave chose the office. The shops were "ugly." Unhappily, much of the good, the useful and the necessary was being classed as "ugly" in this young aesthete's mind, and worse, he was finding himself uncomfortable in the presence of an increasing number of normal, even practically essential conditions. This gifted and promising young man was at odds with reality. He refused to accept reality as real. For him in beauty of line and color and sound, in beauty of thought and expression, only, was the truth. He suffered in other surroundings. He had become aesthetically hypersensitive. And of all reality's ruthlessness, what was less tolerable than monotony? What less capable of leading a man to the heights than the eternal grind of the office?

Even Adelaide and the baby bored him at times. Young Scott could do anything well to which he gave effort. And his father was considering giving him a raise, when at the end of six months he disappeared. The second day after, the distraught wife received a message from New York. He was all right, and would be home next week. The father, however, had to honor another draft before his son could square accounts and purchase a return ticket. This was the first of his retreats from the grim battle-front of reality. Six months seemed the limit of his capacity to face a work-a-day life. He read much, and of the best. He took up Italian alone and soon read it easily. When at home his chief excesses were books-but the Scott table was amply supplied, and in view of his inactive physical habits we realize that Dave was a high liver.

Adelaide had proven a most dutiful daughter-in-law, and with the baby long kept the headsman's ax from descending. But even their restraining power had its limitations. The irk of that "godless" office was being more and more poorly met by Dave. Five times during the fourth year he took ungranted periods of relaxation. The last time the usual draft was not paid. He unwisely signed a check, badly overdrawing his private account. His father seemed waiting for such an opportunity, and took drastic action. Under an old law, he had his son apprehended as a spend thrift, and so adjudged, deprived of his rights and made ward of a guardian. A young physician was made deputy in charge of his person--a man chosen, apparently, with much care. It was to be his business to teach this wealthy man's son to work with his hands and to live on a stipulated sum. There is no question that immediate good followed these aggressive tactics, and in the personality of his companion-guardian he found much that was wholesome. A sturdy character was the doctor, who had fought his way through poverty to a liberal education, and was entering a special study of nervous disorders. His good theoretical training was planted in a rich soil of common-sense. For three months they worked on a farm, shoulder to shoulder. The two men became friends, a most helpful friendship for Dave, whose admiration for the young doctor had proven a path which led him, for the first time, to a realization of the hidden beauties in a life of overcoming, and this lies close to the nobility of the love of work.

Dave was accepting his need for the bitter medicine which was being administered. He had forgiven Adelaide who sided with his father and, for the first time, had written, acknowledging some of his past failures. He wanted some books. He needed clothes. The orders given the doctor had been rigid as to spending-money and diversions. The determined father disapproved the expense account. Another man was sent to relieve the doctor-companion-a man who could be depended upon to carry out the letter of the father's law. Rebellion, fierce--and it seemed, righteous--flamed forth in Dave Scott's soul. He was doing his best. He was working as he never had worked before. He had seen his need--he had the vision of self-mastery. All this, and more he had seriously confided to the man his father, through the court, had placed over him. Without a word of explanation he was again to be turned over to the custody of a stranger. Was he a child or a chattel? Was he mentally irresponsible that he should be thus transferred from one hand to another without a hearing? He wired his protests, and received in return an assurance that he would accept his new custodian or be cut off without a cent. In that hour the real character of David Scott was born. He consulted an attorney and learned the limited power of his guardians. Outside of Ohio he was legally free. He pawned some of his few belongings. Adelaide and the child were financially cared for. Over night he left the State. He would be a man, penniless, rather than the chattel-son of a millionaire!

The United States had just entered the Great War. The Marines were being recruited everywhere for "early over-seas service," and Dave Scott, the aesthetic, volunteered as a "buck-private." Few got over as fast as they wished. It was six months for Dave at Paris Island. There were few in the ranks of his mental ability, and physically he became as hard as the toughest. He was soon a corporal and later a sergeant. And he worked. He met the roughest of camp duties, at first with set jaw and revolting senses, later with a grim smile; finally, and then the emancipation, with a sense of the closeness of man to man in mankind's work. And the men began turning to him, and as he sweated with them he learned to discern the manliness in the crudest of them. He went across at the end of six months, to France. He was a replacement in the Sixth.

The French line had been beaten thin as gold-foil. If it broke, Paris was at the mercy of the Hun. Then eight thousand of Uncle Sam's Marines were thrown in where the line was thinnest and the pressure heaviest. Sharp-shooters, expert marksmen, were most of them. The enemy was now in the open. They had not before met riflemen who boldly stood up and coolly killed at one thousand yards. Crested German helmets made superb targets, and the officers bit the dust disastrously. At the end of three days, six thousand of these eight thousand Marines were dead or casuals. But the tide of the Great War was turned-and Dave Scott was one of the immortals who forced the flood back upon the Rhine. What miracle was it that shielded that ever-smiling white face, crowned with its flaming shock, from the storm of lead and death? With the fate of nations trembling in the balance, who can know the part his blue eyes, now true as steel, played in the great decision as, hour after hour with deadly precision, he turned his hand to slaughter? Five times the gun he was using became too hot and was replaced by that of a dead comrade. After those three days at Chateau-Thierry, no mortal could question that Dave Scott had forsworn aesthetics; that he was a demon of reality. Later he saw service on the Champagne front, and then was invalided home.

It was a chastened father, a magnificently proud father, who was the first to greet him. For the time he was unable to put into words the honor he had for the son whom, so few months before, he considered worthless. "It's all past now, Dave. That past we won't speak of again. I've arranged for your discharge. You'll be home to stay, inside of a month."

Dave's answer, probably more than any act in battle, proved that his character had been remade: "No, Father, I have enlisted for four years. I belong to the Marines till my time is up. I owe it to you, to Adelaide, to the boy, to myself, to prove that I can be the man in peace that I have tried to be in training-camp and in France. I know I can face reality when spurred by excitement. I have yet to prove that I can face the monotony of two years and a half of routine service."

CHAPTER XXII

FINDING THE VICTORIOUS SELF

The victorious soul counts life as a gift which, far from growing darker and more dreary as the sun falls into the west, may daily become more rich and beautiful and worthy. To the soul victorious our span of years is not menaced by misfortune and misery, is not degraded by bitterness, discord and hatred, but hourly thrills with the realization that the worst which life may bring but challenges the divine within to masterful assertion. And the soul victorious has risen unscathed--glorified--above every attack of fate.

Mrs. Herman Judson was a sight to make the gods weep. With features more than usually attractive, softened by a halo of waving, silvery hair, she was but a mushy bog of misery. It was three P. M.; she had just been carried downstairs, and in spite of the usual host of apprehension, with some added new ones for to-day, no slightest accident had marred the perilous trip from her front bedroom to the living-room below; still everything and everybody, save old Dr. Bond, was in a flutter. Tension and apprehension marked the faces and actions of all. Not till the last of six propping, easing, supporting pillows had been adjusted; till hot-water bottles were in near contact with two "freezing" ankles; till her shoulder-shawl had been taken off--a twist straightened out--and accurately replaced; till the room, already ventilated to a preordered nicety of temperature, had a door opened and both windows closed; not till the screen had been moved twice to modify the "glare" of the lights, and to protect from possible "draughts"; not until the "Sunset Scene from Venice" had been turned face to the wall so the reflection from its glass wouldn't make her "eyes run cold water"; and finally, not until ten drops from the bottle labeled "For spinal pain" had been taken, and five minutes spent by her niece, fanning so very gently, "so as not to smother my breath"--not till this formidable contribution to the pitiful slavery of petted sensations had been slavishly offered, could the invalid find strength to greet her childhood playmate, quiet, observing, charitable Dr. Willard Bond.

Twice a day for many months the household held its breath while this moving-down, and later moving-back (and to-day's was an uncomplicated, unusually peaceable one), was being accomplished. "Held its breath," is really not quite accurate, for Ben, the colored butler, and 'Lissie, the colored cook, found much reason for strenuous respiration, as Mrs. Judson and her rocker, with pillows, blankets and the ever present afghan, weighed two hundred and eight pounds-one hundred and eighty pounds of woman, twenty-eight pounds of accessories! And Ben and 'Lissie were the ones who logically deserved fanning and attention to ventilation, especially after the seven P. M. trip back.

And they were always so solemn, so tensifyingly solemn, these risky journeys up and down. The niece, Irma, carried the hot-water bottles, the extra blankets and the fan. The nurse had the medicine-box and a small tray with water-glasses--for when things went wrong, the cavalcade must stop and some of the "Heart-weakness drops" be given, or some whiffs taken from the pungent "For tightness of breath" bottle, before further progress was safe.

Mrs. Judson knew her symptoms so well. There were eighteen of special importance; and Dr. Cummings, the successful young surgeon, a far-away relative-by-marriage, had, in all seriousness, prescribed eighteen lotions, elixirs, powders, pills and potions, to meet each of the eighteen varied symptoms. Nine months ago this progressively developing invalidism of twenty years had culminated in what Dr. Cummings suspected to be a severe gall-stone attack. A few days later, when his sensitive patient was measurably relieved, he had told her his fears and suggested a possible operation. Within two minutes Mrs. Judson was faint and chilling. Since then the doctor, the nurse, the niece, not to forget Ben and 'Lissie, had labored without ceasing to prevent a return of the "awful gall-stone attacks," and, with the Lord's help, to get Mrs. Judson "strong enough for an operation." But progress was dishearteningly slow. Every mention of "operation" seemed to make their patient worse. And now for over eight months she had not walked a step and had been an hourly care.

For the first time since the beginning of the gall-stone trouble, Dr. Cummings was going to be away for two weeks, and he, with Dr. Bond, had witnessed the downstairs trip in anticipation of a conference. Dr. Bond lived but two doors away, and as he had retired from active practice, could always respond to a call if needed. Moreover, it had been discovered that he was a neighbor-playmate of Mrs. Judson during her girlhood. He had but recently come to Detroit from their old home in Charlestown, under the shadow of

Bunker Hill monument, about which they had often played as children. Dr. Bond had lived there alone for many years following his wife's death, and had now come to make a home with his successful son. He was giving his time, and he felt the best year of his life, writing a series of chapters on "Our Nerves and Our Morals." He had never been a specialist, claiming only to be a family- doctor. But for over thirty years he had been ministering most wisely to the ills of the soul as well as of the body. A large, compelling sympathy he gave his patients. He saw their ills. He felt their fears. He sensed their sorrows. He understood their weaknesses. He looked beyond the manifest ailments of flesh and blood. His fine discernment revealed the obscure sicknesses which affect hearts and souls. And his rational sympathies penetrated with the deftness and beneficence of the surgeon's scalpel. He stood for that type of man whom God has raised up to help frail and needing human-kind in body, mind and spirit.

"Sixty years is a long time to pass between meetings, isn't it?" said Dr. Bond after Mrs. Judson's needs had severally and successfully been humored, and she was able to note and recognize the old-new doctor's presence and offer a plump, tremulous hand in greeting.

"You don't know how nearly you have missed seeing me," she replied. "I have been on the verge for months, but Dr. Cummings has been able to pull me through. You see, he knows all my dangers, and has given me the best medicines that medical science knows for each of them. Have him tell you about it, Dr. Bond. I do hope nothing will happen while he's gone." Dr. Bond replied that he was sure, with Dr. Cummings' advice and the nurse's and the niece's help and understanding, there would be no danger; that he was so near he would come in each afternoon and they could talk about the old days and the old childhood friends around Boston. "I hope so," Mrs. Judson replied, "but you know I can't talk long. But do come every day. I'll feel safer, I'm sure. And promise me that you won't delay a minute if I send for you for my gall-stones. If they get started, I die a thousand deaths."

"I shall come at once, you may be sure, but tell the nurse to put those gall-stones to bed at ten p. m., because you and I are too old to be spreeing around during sleeping hours."

But Mrs. Judson couldn't find a ghost of a smile for this pleasantry. In fact, her look of alarm caused Dr. Bond to add, "Don't fear, Mrs. Judson, I can still dress in five minutes and will promise faithfully to come at any hour."

The two physicians left the room together. Thirty-five and sixty-five they were, both earnest, capable, honest men, one a master of modern medical science, the elder a thoroughly equipped physician, and a deep student of humanity.

"I am very glad you are going to see my aunt. For months I have wished to call in a consultant, but she has always refused. I know much of her trouble is nervous, and you know how little time most of us have to study nervousness, and I am sure you will see clearly much which has been rather hazy to me. I think you were concealing a laugh when they gave her the 'Spinal-pain drops,' and frankly, there is very little that has much strength in all those pills and powders I've given her. I have learned that she gets along very well much of the time when she can anticipate her symptoms and prescribe for herself. In fact, it's about all that the poor old lady has to do these days. I am not absolutely sure, either, about those gall-stones. The symptoms are not classic, but she certainly does suffer, and I have had to give her pretty heavy doses of morphine several times, and then she's wretchedly sick for some days. Believe me, Doctor, I do not feel competent in her case. It's not my line. Find out all you can. Do whatever you feel is best, and you may depend upon my endorsement of any changes you may see fit to make. It will be a God's mercy if you can win her confidence and share the burden of her treatment with me. Of course, she's too old to get well, and I'm afraid if we ever have to operate, there will be a funeral."

Dr. Bond thanked the younger man heartily. He felt his earnestness and honesty, and saw that he had done all he knew to help his patient.

That evening the old doctor's mind spanned the gulf of nearly two generations. He was again a little fellow, and Rhoda Burrows lived across the street. Their mothers were friends; they were playmates. And through the years he had treasured her happy, sunny, beautiful face as an ideal of girlhood perfection. She was older than he, and how she had "big sistered" and "mothered" him! How his little hurts and sorrows had fled before her laughter and caresses! Hundreds and thousands had touched his inner life since Rhoda moved West with her parents, but that gleam of girlhood had remained etched with the clearness of a miniature upon his mind, undimmed by the crowding, jostling throng. Rhoda Burrows, the fairy-child of his boyish dreams, and Mrs. Herman Judson, the acme of self-pitying and self-petting selfishness, the same! It seemed impossible--yet--and here his big charity spoke--all of the choice spirit of the girl cannot have been swallowed up in the sordidness of a selfish, old age. And that same charity breathed upon the physician's soul till his helpful and hopeful interest for this pitiful wreck of wretchedness was aglow. He would give her his best, and he knew that best sometimes wrought wonders.

Dr. Bond first had a conference with the niece, who was pure gold, and who accepted each of her aunt's complaints as a warning which could but disastrously be ignored. But, and this was good to know, he learned that when Aunt Rhoda was better, she was kind and good- hearted. From the nurse, the doctor learned other details, and what was of special significance, that the invalid's appetite rarely flagged-then he saw a reason for her one hundred and eighty pounds; and when he learned that rare broiled beef, or rare roast beef was served the physically inert patient and bountifully eaten twice each day, his understanding became active.

Mrs. Judson's presiding fates were good to her the next week. She would have denied it with the sum total of her vehemence, which incidentally was some sum, but Dr. Bond says it is true. It was after eleven, one night. He was just finishing his day's writing. It was the nurse 'phoning. "I am truly sorry to call you, Doctor, but I've given three doses of the gall-stone medicine, and it always relieves unless a real attack is on. I am sure she is suffering." The old doctor was not surprised. The patient had been doing unusually well for two or three days and had spoken particularly of her better appetite. The doctor's first query, upon reaching the house, related to the details of the evening meal. "No, there was no steak to-night. We had chicken- salad. 'Lissie had tried herself; Mrs. Judson was hungry and asked for a second portion."

Gently, carefully, thoroughly, the suffering woman was examined. There was no doubt that her pain was severe, but in conclusion, the old doctor did doubt decidedly the presence of gall-stones. He believed it to be duodenal colic. "I don't wish to give you a hypodermic," he told her. "I know it will relieve you quickly to-night, but it will set you back several days. I am going to ask you to be patient, and to take an unpleasant dose, and I think the nurse and I can relieve you completely within two hours, and you will be little the worse; in fact, you may be better, to-morrow."

"She won't take it," the nurse said, as the doctor called her from the room. "Dr. Cummings suggested it once, and she held it against him for weeks. She said her mother whipped her when she was a child and then couldn't make her swallow it."

"You will fix it as I tell you, then bring it in to me," the Doctor replied. Dubiously the nurse carried out the order. She thanked her stars that the Doctor, not she, was to give it. Yet it looked very nice when she brought it into the sick-room, redolent with lemon and peppermint.

"Think of this, Mrs. Judson, as your best friend to-night in all the realm of medicine. Take it with my belief that it is to prove the cure of your gall-stones. It is not nice. It's not easy to swallow. Don't sip it. Take it all at a gulp."

But she sipped it. And she screamed, not a scream of pain, but of rage, of violated dignity-insulted-outraged. "Castor oil! I'll die first. Why, that stuff isn't fit to give an animal. Are you trying to kill me I Oh, you old fogy! I knew something would happen when I let Dr. Cummings go. I wouldn't give such stuff to a sick cat."

All symptoms of pain seemed gone for the time. Generous as he was, the old Doctor stiffened in the face of her tirade, yet with dignity, replied: "You are refusing a real help. I speak from long experience. I can give you nothing else till you have taken this."

"Then go!" she snapped out. But the "o-o-o" was prolonged into a wail as a particularly pernicious jab in the midst of her duodenum-"a providential thrust," Dr. Bond said--doubled her up, if rotundity can be said to double. The Doctor was obdurate. Colic was trumps--and won!

The first dose did not meet a hospitable reception, but another was promptly given. Then other nicer things were done and the Doctor was home and the patient comfortably asleep soon after one. The next day's conference between the two was strictly professional, nor was there much thawing till the third day after. Mrs. Judson's ire must have been of Celtic origin, for it was not long-lived.

The following Sunday afternoon seemed propitious for the beneficent work of the soul-doctor. The whole family had told Mrs. Judson how much better she was looking-the Doctor had kept her on soft diet since her attack. "You have told me so little of yourself," said Dr. Bond. "I only know that sorrow came." He then told her of herself as she had lived in his memory. She had forgotten the beauty of her childhood. The Doctor brought back the picture in tones which could stand only for high reverence. She felt he wanted to know, and she knew she wanted to tell. So for two hours they sat, hand in hand, as in their childhood, and he heard of her father's moderate success as an editorial writer after he came West when she was nine, of their comfortable home in Detroit, how well she had done in school, of her early ability as a teacher, of her election as super-intendent of the St. Claire Academy for Girls when she was twenty-five, of her marriage to Herman Judson, a childless widower fifteen years her senior, before she was thirty, of their very happy home, of her own little girl and how she grew into womanhood, of her daughter's marriage, and then of tier little girl, and how wonderful it was to be a grandmother before she was fifty!

Then it was "Nurse, the bottle for 'Tightness of breath'... I don't see how I can tell it. You can't know. Nobody can. It was never the same for any one else. The train went through a bridge, and they were all three killed, my husband, my only girl, the darling grandchild. God turned His face away that night they brought them home. I've never seen Him since. I've never looked for Him since. I don't see how I kept my mind. Something snapped inside. I couldn't go to the funeral, and while I brought my sister home to live with me, and after she died, have done the best I could to raise Irma, her child, and Irma's tried, I know, to be a daughter to me, yet I've always been so lonely, so wretched and miserable and sick. I haven't anything to live for-but I'm afraid to die."

Then began the cheapening catalog of the nearly twenty years of illness, her weak and sensitive spine, her constant difficulty in breathing, and the eternal thumping of her heart. And on and on, the list so old to Dr. Bond's ears, so commonly heard in the experience of helpers of the nervous sick-as usual to the nerve-specialist as the inflamed appendix to the modern surgeon--yet in the mind of every nerve-sufferer so unique, so individual, so different. But of all the long, two-hour story, one short sentence stood out, eloquent in the doctor's mind, "I haven't anything to live for, yet I'm afraid to die." He gently thanked her. He had felt with her in the recital of her great sorrow, and she knew he had suffered in her suffering. "You can get well. You can find something worth living for, and you can lose your fear of death, if you will pay the price." For the moment she misunderstood.

"Why, Doctor, I would gladly give thousands for health."

Again, gently, "Your dollars are worthless. You are poor in the gold which will buy your restoration. I shall tell you about it Wednesday if you want to know."

On both Monday and Tuesday visits her curiosity prompted her to refer to the great cure Dr. Bond mentioned. But it was Wednesday afternoon before he spoke seriously.

"You were very ill last week--such illnesses have frequently proved fatal to life, when ignorantly managed. But as I see you to-day, knowing your radiant childhood, and the good fortune which was yours for years, and the heart-tearing shock which came so cruelly, I see a sickness more dire and fatal than any for which you have ever yet been treated. The beauty and youth and charity of your spirit are mortally ill. I see your soul an emaciated remnant, a skeleton of its possible self. It threatens to die before your body. Selfish sorrow has infected and permeated your once lovely, better self, and to-day you have no true goodness left. You are good to others that they may be better to you. You are generous with your means-a generosity which costs you no sacrifice, that you may buy back the generosity without which you could not live. Four useful lives are emptying the best of their strength, ability and love into years of service that you may know a poor, low-grade, selfish, physical comfort. You are taking from them and others consideration, self-sacrifice, loyalty, unstinted devotion, and giving in return only ungrateful dollars. You are rich in these, but poorer than Lazarus in the least of the qualities which make life worth living a day, which keep Death from being a haunting terror. You have not one physical symptom of your endless catalog which cannot be removed if you meet the blessings half-way which discomforts offer."

It couldn't have been what Dr. Bond said--it must have been what he was himself that made those unwelcome, humiliating truths carry conviction, win confidence, and waken hope. Possibly his last sentence helped her decision-- his serious confidence in his ability to remove those terrifying, ever impending threats of physical anguish. At any rate, she gave her promise-for six months she would implicitly follow his instruction, with the understanding that if she did not see herself better at the end of four months, she was to be released from further treatment.

It would be a long story, a story of remarkable medical finesse; it would be describing the work of an artist--for such was Dr. Bond as he turned bodies from sickness to health and souls from perdition to salvation. But victory came! In six weeks, the invalid was walking. In six months she was walking three miles a day. She was eating, bathing, sleeping and working more like a woman under sixty than one nearing seventy. She spent the summer with the doctor's people in their bungalow on Lake Huron. She now gave of her means thoughtfully, with growing unselfishness, and soon after she began to look up and out there came the peace within, so long a stranger. And she told Dr. Bond, simply, one day, that God had come back to her, and he as simply replied: "You have come back to God."

That winter, Dr. Bond spent in the East. One day the expressman brought a package--some books he had always loved, in remarkable bindings, and this note:

"My best Friend:

"To-day I am seventy. I haven't been so young since sorrow was sent to prove me, nor more happy since I nursed your hurt arm when we were children. I walked down town, two miles you know, and back, and a mile in the stores, I am sure, to find these books you love, in bindings worthy your better enjoyment of them. All that you have promised has come to me. God bless you!"

CHAPTER XXIII

THE TRIUMPH OF HARMONY

When man "conceives his superpower, his miraculous power to meet disaster, and in it to find profit; to face defeat after defeat and therein acquire faith in his own permanence; to live for years within a frail, defective body, with a mind unable to respond to the promptings of ambition and inspiration, and thereby take on the greatness of gentleness-the conviction comes clear, a conviction which will not comfortably stay put aside, that life is intended to develop a noble self."

What could be more beautiful to senses that thrill with love than this pink-cheeked, azure-eyed babe, whose golden ringlets promise the glorious crown, the unfading beauty of her womanhood? She was hardly a month old, yet she seemed to understand--Mammy Lou said she did-that she must look her "beau'fulest"; so when her father came and bent over her little crib, she smiled, then coyly ducked her wobbly head, to smile again at Mother, the dear mother who only to-day had been allowed by the doctor to sit up for an hour. Mammy Lou must have been right, for there Baby lay playing with her fingers and the disappointed pink ribbons of her booties, while, now and then, when the discussion was specially serious, she would look soberly at her earnest-faced parents till they both would notice, and laugh. Then her little understanding smile-and some more play. It was an important conference. Considerations affecting Baby's future were in the balance, and, as she gave such perfect attention and never interrupted, and insisted on every one keeping good-natured, Mammy Lou's assertion that "Dat lil' sweetness' stood every word her pa an' ma said. She knew dey's findin' her a name," cannot be successfully disputed.

The Southards had been married twelve years. Georgia was eight, and Etta five. It must be a boy--one who would pass on the Southard name and traditions. The first Earl of Minto had contributed some nobleness of blood to the Southard stock, and the father had set his heart on a boy who should feel the double inspiration of "Minto Southard," to help make him fine and great.

A "girl"! And business took the father away for a fortnight. It was rumored that he drowned his disappointment in Charleston-but not in the Bay. He did not fully realize that the brave wife was gravely ill, until his return. Then he was devoted and tender. They had made no plans for a little girl; so she was nearly a month old and was still being called "Sweetness" by Mammy Lou, and "The Baby" by others, and to-day, while Mother first sat up, her name was to be decided.

"Why, Father, dear, no girl was ever called that. I think it would be all right for a boy, but she's such a dainty little thing, and I'm sure it will always seem odd to her."

"What would you like better, Mater? I don't wish to contend or to be unduly insistent, but you know I have looked forward to having the Earl's name in the family, and, personally, I think it has the attraction of uniqueness, as well as the flavor of distinction. Then, you remember, you suggested the names for the other girls. I know you are thinking of her future and fear an odd name may make her unhappy, some time. But we can, we should, teach her to be proud of so distinguished an association. My personal desire is very strong, and I can't think of any other name which will satisfy me nearly as well."

Just then Baby looked at her mother, smiled and gurgled something which was intelligible to mother-ears, and the wife's hand slipped into the husband's, and the baby was named Minta Southard.

Where could a new baby have found a more perfect setting for her childhood and girlhood? The plantation lay on both sides of the Catawba River-fresh and crystal clear those days, as it sped down from mountains to sea-fertile, fruitful acres there were, which never failed to bring forth manyfold. Three times in as many generations, the Manor House, as the rambling southern home had always been called, had been enlarged, but nothing was ever done which lessened the dignity lent by its fine colonial portico, the artistic columns of which could be seen miles down the river-road. The Manor House was good to see in its rare setting of stately water-oaks, now in their full maturity.

For four years little Minta thrived and gave promise of bringing many joys to this home which knew no shadow but the father's periodic "business trips" to Charleston. Mammy Lou was her slave, and even Georgia, who had her own way so much that she was far from unselfish, asked, at times, to "take care" of her dainty sister, and would let her play with some of her things without protest. Then the fever! "Typhoid," the doctor said, "affecting her brain." Father, Mother and Mammy Lou took turns being with her those long, hot weeks, when it forgot to rain and the refreshing sea-breeze was cruelly withheld. Doctors from Charlotte, doctors from Charleston and doctors from Atlanta came, to look grave, to shake their learned heads, and to sadly leave, offering no hopeful change in treatment. The fever was prolonged over five weeks, and the child seemed more lifeless each day as it left her drained and damaged--drained and damaged for life it proved. So slowly her shadowy form gained, that a single week was too short to evidence improvement. Six months, and she was not yet walking. One year, and she was still fragile. Then, in a month, normal childhood apparently slipped back, and she began to play and be merry.

Of course "Sweetness" was spoiled--and an autocrat she was, her mother, only, denying herself the indulgence of being her subject. Mother, however, was lovingly tactful, and exercised the discipline she believed necessary for her child's good most wisely. And Mother's memory has ever remained a hallowed one. Mammy Lou did much to discredit all of the mother's conscientious care. For so long the poor child "couldn't eat no thin'," and when at last Minta's appetite returned, her loving black nurse would give her anything she wanted, and if the fever hadn't hopelessly damaged the little one's digestive glands, Mammy Lou's unfailing "l'il snacks for her honey-chile" would have completed the wreckage. At first the trouble was not noticed. Minta rarely spoke of suffering. She would be found lying with her face from the light, and would always reply that she was "tired playing," sometimes only, "my head hurts." The parents thought she did play too hard, for she was developing into an intense little miss, who entered into whatever she was doing with more than blue-eyed zest, those blue eyes which snapped blue-black when her will was crossed.

The girls all had their early teaching at home, so when Minta was thirteen, Miss Allison came from Washington to spend a year, as tutor, to prepare her for school the next fall. That was the year Georgia ran away. She had been visiting in Savannah several weeks, when she disappeared, leaving a hurried note to her friends, stating that she would write her people from New York, and begging them not to worry about her. The note from New York was thoughtlessly written. She was probably frightened by what she had done. She was safe in New York with Randolph, where they would be for ten days. She was sorry. Would they forgive her? She knew she had done wrong. Write her at --- East Fourteenth Street, where they were boarding.

The outraged father called the two girls and their mother into his office, and read them Georgia's letter, then tore it into bits. "Your sister's name is never to be mentioned again in this house. She has brought the first dishonor to the Southard name in America. She is disowned, and may she be swallowed up in her own disgrace."

Nothing had ever so impressed Minta as her father's face that day. A primitive savagery spoke, intensified by the refinements of Cavalier blood. No one dared utter a word of protest. He was implacable as adamant, they all knew. Mr. Southard was never the same. Some of his genial tenderness was lost forever, and the family lived on with the unmentionable name ever before them, like a grave which was never to be filled. The father was away much more the following year. He never drank at home. And, after his death, it was found that he had gambled away many thousands-all of Georgia's part. Thus a father's pride of family met a daughter's impulse.

The little mother, never strong, always patient and devoted and lovable, seemed unable to rise above the shame and the sorrow of it all, and could give less and less to Minta, who now found in Miss Allison and Mammy Lou her most potent influences. Miss Allison was worthy the responsibility and probably did much to decide the girl's future. She had studied art, and had hoped to spend years abroad. Financial disappointments had made this impossible. But her imaginative pupil loved the art of which she spoke so often, and begged to be taught to sketch. She early showed unusual skill and the promise of talent; still the father would not consider her going North with Miss Allison to school. Yet the seeds had been sown and an artist she was to be. But the cost!

Two years she spent at Converse College. During the second summer-vacation her father died, and as her mother's heart was gradually weakening, Minta stayed at home the following year. A few weeks before the dear mother slipped away, she talked with Minta about the older sister, dutifully avoiding the mention of her name. "I have never felt right about the way we treated her," she said. "Some time when you are older, won't you try to find her and help her?"

The Cavalier was in the younger daughter too. "I certainly think she has caused unhappiness enough. She made our home a different place, and she shortened Father's life. I can't forgive her."

"But, Daughter, we don't know. There may have been some mistake."

Minta was decided. "She no longer belongs to the Southard family. Father was right."

The mother did not insist, and only said, "She, too, is my child. She is of your blood. We should forgive."

Her mother was with her but a few weeks after this conversation. And, within two months after her funeral, an attack of pneumonia robbed Minta's already frail body of strength which might have come at that developing age. Much of the next eighteen months she spent in bed. It was then decided that she consult a friend of her father's, a city physician. Unfortunately, this ambitious surgeon had been but a convivial friend. His professional development had reached only the "operation" stage. Surgery to him was a panacea, and the operation, which he promised to be her saving, was to be her tragedy. She did not know till two years later that she had been robbed of her birthright. Her headaches, far from being helped, were even worse, now blinding and exhausting. She at last went East to a world-renowned specialist who undid, as far as his great skill could, the damage of the first operation, and who, great man that he was, had time not only to operate but to comprehend. His cultivated instincts led him directly to an intimacy with his patient's idealisms, and he was one to whom every right-souled sufferer could trust his deepest confidence without reserve.

"I fear, little girl, your ambitions are only for those of unquestioned strength. You are but a pigmy. Certain organs, essential to the conversion of food into energy, were injured beyond all repair in your first illness. Other damage which neither time nor skill can make good was inflicted by your first operation. Your eyes are entirely inadequate for the merciless exactions of a life of art. You are at best but a delicate hot-house plant-beyond human power to develop into sufficient hardiness to be transplanted into the world of Bohemia, or into much of any world save a sheltered one. You can never be more than a semi-invalid."

This sentence the great doctor pronounced only after his own opinion had been re-enforced by a conference of experts. And every word was true, as far as he and the experts had investigated.

But there was the spirit of a Cavalier with which they had not reckoned. "I'll not have it so. Life, the life that you give me, isn't worth living. I shall have my two years in Europe with my art, if it takes all those other years you say I can have by saving myself."

And she had them! One year first in New York in preparation, then two years in Rome. Three weeks she worked; one week she suffered. And how wonderfully she did suffer! She had been warned of the danger of drug- relief. And when doctors came and began filling their hypodermic syringes, her indignation blazed up. "If that's all you have for me, you needn't come. I could give that to myself." She learned that quiet and darkness, and, it seemed, fasting, dulled the edge of the pain and shortened its duration, and that nothing else did as much.

There was another art student in Rome-a fine, poor American who, too, was studying art because he loved it. How they could have helped each other! They both knew it. It was as natural as life, after they had worked together a few months, for him to ask if she could wait while he earned, and made a name. She knew that waiting was not necessary; that she had plenty for them both and that she could help him, as few others, to more quickly win the fame which he was sure to attain. And she knew, too, that she could not so love another-there was never a doubt of that. But this time love was bitterly cruel. It came in all its affection and beauty only to sear and rend. She "must not marry," the great surgeon had told her. So gently and fatherly he had said it, that she did not realize its full import till now. Husbandless, childless, a chronic, incurable sufferer, she must tread the wine- press alone!

The man had gone. She could give him no reason. She could not remember what she said to him. The world went black, and consciousness fled. For weeks she lay in an Italian hospital. Etta and her husband came, and the only rational words they could hear were her pleadings to be taken back to Dr. Kingsley.

Somehow the trip was made. But it was a desperately sick girl, the mere shell of a life, that they returned to America. It was weeks before she realized where she was and other weeks before she was able to tell Dr. Kingsley so that he could understand it all--not only of sorrow's final revelation, but this time, what she had not mentioned before, of Georgia--the family disgrace. She did not know the wonderful power of Christian counsel and ideals to save from the so- often misinterpreted sufferings of wrong spiritual adjustments. She had not realized the healing power of the love of God expressed in the lives of good men and women, and how it can sweeten the bitterness and dissipate even the paralyzing loneliness of an impossible human love.

Dr. Kingsley's eyes had welled with tears when she told the story of Georgia. How impellingly gentle was his voice when he said, "You'll forgive her now, I know." Forgive her! What else to do, when he made it so noble and beautiful and right. So when she was strong enough, she began looking for the sister who had so complicated the years, and, through an old school-friend, traced her to a little flat. And it was even as her mother had thought. Georgia had married, "beneath the family," she told Minta, the Georgia who was too proud to ever write again. She was living in Brooklyn, the wife of Randolph, an assistant engineer on an ocean steamship. And Etta came to visit Georgia, and a great load, a load of which she had, through the years, been unconscious, slipped away as Minta let go her enmity. "In all things," she said to Dr. Kingsley, "I am your obedient patient-all things but one. I will work, and I shall work."

And she does work. No one understands how. Seventy-odd pounds of frailty, with eyes which are ever resentful of the use to which she puts them; with the recurrence of suffering which wrings every ounce of physical strength, which for days holds her mind writhing as on the rack, which tortures her to physical and mental surrender, but which, through the lengthening years, has been impotent to daunt her regal spirit.

And she gives, gives on through the days of relative comfort, gives of her cheer which comes from, no one knows where; gives, spontaneously, kindness which has multiplied her lovers, both men and women; and gives of her ability which is unquestioned. There are a few publishers who know her skill. There is a touch of pathos in all she draws, pathos-never bitterness, never ugliness-always the breath of beauty.

Minta Southard, hopelessly defective in what we call health, has triumphed through the harmony of a brave adjustment to her pitiless limitations-a harmony realized by few, even though rich, in resource of mind, powerful, in reserve of body.

Can we ignore the omnipotence of the spiritual?

###

www.ingramcontent.com/pod-product-compliance
Lightning Source LLC
Chambersburg PA
CBHW070858180526
45168CB00005B/1870